The Magic Teaspoon

Most Berkley Books are available at special quantity discounts for bulk purchases for sales promotions, premiums, fund-raising, or educational use. Special books, or book excerpts, can also be created to fit specific needs.

For details, write: Special Markets, The Berkley Publishing Group, 375 Hudson Street, New York, New York 10014.

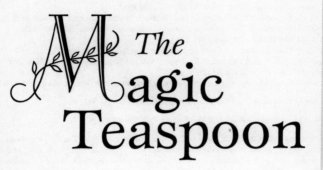

The Magic Teaspoon

*Transform Your Meals
with the Power of
Healing Herbs and Spices*

Victoria Zak

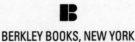

BERKLEY BOOKS, NEW YORK

THE BERKLEY PUBLISHING GROUP
Published by the Penguin Group
Penguin Group (USA) Inc.
375 Hudson Street, New York, New York 10014, USA
Penguin Group (Canada), 90 Eglinton Avenue East, Suite 700, Toronto, Ontario M4P 2Y3, Canada
(a division of Pearson Penguin Canada Inc.)
Penguin Books Ltd., 80 Strand, London WC2R 0RL, England
Penguin Group Ireland, 25 St. Stephen's Green, Dublin 2, Ireland (a division of Penguin Books Ltd.)
Penguin Group (Australia), 250 Camberwell Road, Camberwell, Victoria 3124, Australia
(a division of Pearson Australia Group Pty. Ltd.)
Penugin Books India Pvt. Ltd., 11 Community Centre, Panchsheel Park, New Delhi—110 017, India
Penguin Group (NZ), Cnr. Airborne and Rosedale Roads, Albany, Auckland 1310, New Zealand
(a division of Pearson New Zealand Ltd.)
Penguin Books (South Africa) (Pty.) Ltd., 24 Sturdee Avenue, Rosebank, Johannesburg 2196, South Africa

Penguin Books Ltd., Registered Offices: 80 Strand, London WC2R 0RL, England

This book is an original publication of The Berkley Publishing Group.

Copyright © 2006 by Victoria Zak
Cover design by Rita Frangie
Cover photo by axb group
Text design by Tiffany Estreicher

PRINTING HISTORY
Berkley trade paperback edition / June 2006

Library of Congress Cataloging-in-Publication Data

Zak, Victoria.
    The magic teaspoon : transform your meals with the power of healing herbs and spices / by Victoria Zak.
        p. cm.
    Includes bibliographical references and index.
    ISBN 0-425-20983-0
    1. Herbs—Therapeutic use.   2. Spices—Therapeutic use.   I. Title

RM666.H33Z342   2006
615'.321—dc22

                                                                                          2006042692

PRINTED IN THE UNITED STATES OF AMERICA

10   9   8   7   6   5   4   3   2   1

ACKNOWLEDGMENTS

I'd like to thank Sally McMillan and Christine Zika, and the following people for their support: Don Axinn, Stacey Chase, Sarah Cressy, Jane Early, Katie and Mike Frassinelli, Steve Halpert, Katherine Hogan, Sheila Joslin, Jennifer Keen, Carole Missaggia, Linda Payne, Margaret Perkins, Judith Podell, and Judy and Cliff Wagner.

Special Acknowledgment
Several friends shared their favorite recipes with me and were very good-natured about letting me adapt them to the high-energy eating style of *The Magic Teaspoon*, if necessary. Others gave me family recipes that had been handed down through generations to share with you, and many were also taste testers for my recipes. We talked endlessly about herbs, spices, and minute details that can help to make recipes easy to understand and easy to follow by everyone. Their encouragement kept me inspired. The following people helped to make *The Magic Teaspoon* special: Betty Badavis, Linda Bell, Bill and Jennifer Bowman, Cris Carlin, Michael Dowling, Kim Dustin, Rose Fidel, Miriam Georgaroudakis, Tasha Halpert, Karen Henderson, Faye Kalmbach, Laura Kennedy, Vivian Kolovos, Marie Lucking, Sally McMillan, Victoria Medaglia, Martha Oldham, Lora Peers, Barbara Reed, Phil Scheidt, Robert Vesprini, and Kathy Zak.

Working with herbs and spices is also a tribute to all of the herbalists, gardeners, and historians who have kept this spirit of the herbs and spices alive through generations. To contact the author: victoriazak2001@yahoo.com.

To Tasha Halpert, whose love for herbs, holistic cooking style, and unlimited grace changed the way I cook and the way I look at life. Thank you, Tasha. Your friendship is a great gift.

CONTENTS

Part I

The Magic Teaspoon Herbs & Spices

   The legends and lore of the herbs and spices come to life in your kitchen. In an alphabetical guide from allspice to watercress, you'll find stories of the herbs and spices in history, their health profiles and culinary uses, and you'll travel to gardens of the world for inspiration.

   This chart is the first of its kind to identify the vital health benefits of the herbs and spices for cooking in one easy reference guide. It includes natural antioxidants, anti-inflammatories, antacids, antibiotics, antidepressants, digestive aids, diabetes fighters, cancer fighters, cholesterol reducers, and more.

Part II

The Magic Teaspoon Recipes

Health and pleasure combine in energizing recipes to boost your immunity; increase your vitality; reduce inflammation; lower cholesterol; fight diabetes, heart disease, digestive disorders, depression, and free radical damage; and help you burn fat.

More than one hundred recipes are provided for breakfast, lunch, dinner, and snacks that include fabulous herbal purees, soups, sandwiches, sauces, dips, salads and fresh dressings, and healing iced teas. You'll also find easy ways to transform your processed food into healthier fare and gain sugar smarts to help you cut excess sugar without sacrificing sweetness. The power is in your food!

PART I

The Magic Teaspoon Herbs & Spices

CHAPTER 1

INTRODUCTION
An Adventure
in Healing Pleasure

You could be one teaspoon away from a healthier life!

Consider the Mediterranean herb thyme, for instance, and what it might do for your health when you use it in your everyday menu.

Aromatic thyme has a mild antibiotic to strengthen your immunity. It contains a vital antiseptic to cleanse your system. It's antiviral, antibacterial, antifungal, and antimicrobial to combat colds, flu, viruses, and fungal infections, particularly in your respiratory system.

Think of what that can mean when flu season arrives. With thyme in your menu, you're in a less risky position to pick up every seasonal infection, and your system has greater defenses in germ-prone environments like schools, offices, and public buildings where people are sniffling, sneezing, and feverish. If you do get the flu, it's far more likely that you'll experience a milder version of it and recover with greater speed and ease, because you have the infection-fighting defenses of thyme in your menu.

With a flick of your teaspoon, you can add thyme to tuna salad, use thyme in burgers, and sauté vegetables in thyme for a richer taste and greater immune strength. Or you can make mushroom crisps with olive oil and thyme; they take one minute to prepare, and they cook themselves in the oven at high heat in five to eight minutes, for fabulous veggie treats. That's how easy it can be to enhance your health and pleasure in one recipe.

Consider the herb dill, a favored herb in Scandinavian countries. It's a natural stimulant to give you energy, and it's a *nervine*—an herb that soothes your nervous system to reduce anxiety and help you sleep better. It strengthens respiration, opens blood vessels, helps to lower high blood pressure, and calms digestive difficulties. It fights infections and inflammations and eases pain.

One teaspoon of dill in green salad, potato salad, or a sauté for vegetables will increase your defenses against many common diseases. Or you can make Dill Deliverance puree (see chapter 8) to get the power of dill in a puree that can be combined with cottage cheese, sour cream, or yogurt cheese for a dreamy, versatile dip that can also be used as a topping for omelets, fish, and chicken.

And that's only two of the life-enhancing herbs you can add to your everyday menu for your pleasure and health.

The sweet herb basil is a tonic for your adrenal glands, a natural antidepressant, an immune system stimulant, and a powerful infection fighter. Basil is a natural for chicken and fish, vibrant in green salad, and wonderful with tomatoes—wait until you try baked tomatoes drizzled in olive oil and basil, with fresh grated Parmesan. You can enhance your immunity and fight infections, all through pure pleasure.

Cinnamon is an antiseptic spice that fights viruses, bacteria, and fungal infections, including E. coli and candida. It helps to reduce blood pressure, and studies suggest that cinnamon can help to ward off adult-onset diabetes. How can you use cinnamon in your menu for power and satisfaction? Try my Cinnamon Nectar (see chapter 10), a light, creamy blend of sour cream, yogurt, honey, and cinnamon that can be used as a salad dressing or topping for fruit. It's a recipe for pleasure, with the health benefits of cinnamon as a bonus.

Did you know that cayenne pepper is an infection fighter and a pain reliever, and it helps to burn fat?

And that's only five of the herbs and spices that you can use to enhance your health.

You'll find more than forty herbs and spices, and many varieties of peppers, mustards, and blends described in detail in chapter 2, "Nature's Bouquet of Healing Herbs and Spices for Cooking." I also developed a chart for you called "The All-Naturals" to give you a quick reference source for the herbs and spices that are natural antibiotics, natural anti-inflammatories, natural antacids, natural digestive aids, antioxidants, cancer fighters, cholesterol reducers, and more. You can use this guide to target specific herbs and spices for specific health needs.

With a flick of a teaspoon, you can make sauces and salads sing with flavor, but it's not just the flavor you will savor. It's a powerful health menu you can use to defend yourself against seasonal infections, stress and its depleting effects, colds, flu, viruses, and intestinal infections, and you can strengthen your immunity to life-limiting diseases.

Adding Vitality to Processed Foods

We've all been told that eating fresh food is the ideal way to get the best nutrition from our meals, because the nutritional content of fresh food is greater than that of processed food. But it isn't always practical to eat freshly prepared meals in our fast-paced world, with time constraints and budget concerns. If you're like most people who rely on a variety of processed foods for quick-cook standbys— like tomato sauce in jars, pouch pastas, boxed macaroni and cheese, and canned soups—does that mean you have to settle for downsized nutrition? Not if you use a little imagination and lots of herbal energy to drive up the power of processed foods. I've included a guide to help you boost the healing power of your processed foods and take one more step toward enhancing your health.

If you don't use a rich bouquet of herbs and spices to enhance your everyday menu, you'll be surprised to see the health-boosting energy you could be missing. If you're already a lover of herbs and spices, and have a collection of recipes, you'll find a few more delights to inspire you, like One Phenomenal Potato Salad, and Summer in a Bowl—high-energy salads that can be used for main meals or snacks.

Health is inspiring, but so is pleasure. You'll find both in *The Magic Teaspoon* recipes.

Iced Teas for Healing

You can also use your magic teaspoon to take herbs as teas, since the standard dose of tea—even medicinal ones in history—is one teaspoon.

To complete this high-energy eating style, I've included top-notch teas for healing in my signature iced teas to strengthen your immunity, get you through high-stress days, and make you the best that you can be. Consider green tea, if you've been on the run all day, living on take-out snacks, and your diet has suffered for it. One cup of green tea will give you the antioxidants of seven vegetables! This is not to suggest that you should drink green tea instead of eating vegetables, but if you haven't eaten a vegetable all day, green tea can give your body a boost of antioxidant power, and you'll get the benefits of green tea's anticancer virtues as well. Try my recipe for Green Tea Sunrise as an iced tea for your thermos for the office, gym, or traveling. It's an energizer!

Sugar Smarts

If you're a sugar lover, and you tend to rely on high-sugar sodas or fruit drinks for quick energy boosts, you'll find an easy, energizing way to lose 56 teaspoons of sugar from your system in one week, with one iced tea in a thermos. You can lose 224 teaspoons of sugar from your system in one month, reaping remarkable health benefits.

The Magic Teaspoon is designed for real people in the real world, like you and me. We all face stresses in our working lives, with time constraints, budget concerns, and pressures of seasonal vacations, holidays, parties, and events that leave us feeling "under the weather." Does that mean we have to settle for diminished nutrition and meals without a gourmet flavor? Not at all. *The Magic Teaspoon* recipes will show you how to eat for power and pleasure at the same time. Best of all, it's not out of your reach or complicated. All it takes is a flick of your magic teaspoon.

Is There Magic in This Teaspoon?

The teaspoon has a long history as a trusted dose of medicine, dating back thousands of years when herbs and spices were the *only* medicines, grown in gardens around the world, including monastic and royal gardens. The earliest prescriptions by doctors and herbalists were given in doses of one teaspoon, whether the herbs or spices were taken alone or in blends. Doctors, to this day, prescribe teaspoon doses of natural and synthetic medicines as trusted measures—especially for children. Historically, mothers commonly administered a trusted dose of medicine—and the mother has remained a universal symbol of caregiving and healing throughout the ages. Herbs and spices come from Mother Nature, and so . . . this teaspoon comes full circle to your table with a trusted dose of natural support from Mother Nature.

There is one more important aspect of herbs to consider. Herbs, which are often *perceived* as medicines because of their vital healing properties, are in fact foods! The foods we commonly call *vegetables* are actually herbs. The onion is a bulb of an herb, carrots and parsnips are roots of herbs, while celery and asparagus are stems of herbs. Our fruits come from herbal trees, bushes, and plants. Our salad greens are the leaves of herbs, just like rosemary, thyme, and peppermint. Our spices come from dried fruits or powdered roots of herbs that have been used throughout history for both medicines and foods.

Is there magic in this teaspoon? Absolutely! The magic is in your food! The teaspoon is in your hand. All you have to do is use it.

Welcome to *The Magic Teaspoon*—an adventure in healing pleasure. We're going to make a little magic with food.

CHAPTER 2

Nature's Bouquet of Healing Herbs and Spices for Cooking

Legend and lore are the perfumes in the air as we take this journey through herbal gardens of the world. When you pick the leaves of a fresh herb or measure a teaspoon of dried herbs for a recipe, thousands of years of tradition come to life in your kitchen.

Each herb in "Nature's Bouquet of Healing Herbs and Spices for Cooking" has a common name and a Latin name that it has carried through history. The common name can change to accommodate different languages. For instance, *turmeric* in English is called *haldi* in India. But the Latin name remains as a stamp of identity to allow us to distinguish the official medicinal herb from its family members that may look similar and have a similar fragrance, but may not have the same healing virtues or history of use. For instance, there are many varieties of sages, but only *Salvia officinalis* is considered the official medical herb that is sanctioned through its use in history.

The Latin name gives you a reference point to use when you are buying herbs for their healing virtues; you can check the Latin name to verify that you are getting the official herb, not an imitator. In addition, the Latin name is vital when you want to check scientific literature on a specific herb, since scientific studies often use *only* the Latin name. The Latin name can also give you a glimpse into the herb's stature in history. For instance, *salvia* in the Latin name of sage means to "heal."

Some Enchanted Evening in Your Kitchen . . .

Take a minute to feel the texture of a fresh or dried herb or spice in your fingers. Inhale its fragrance, taste a bit on your tongue, and think of the journey the herb or spice has taken to come to your table. Each herb or spice represents the bounty of nature in lands far and near, the care it took to grow and harvest them in season, and the global cooperation it takes to bring each special taste, color, and fragrance to your table—to make a little magic in your kitchen.

ALLSPICE
Seeds of Zest

Pimenta dioica (offinalis)
PART USED: Dried Berries

Picture yourself taking an afternoon walk on the limestone hills of Jamaica, overlooking an azure sea. Just ahead, there is a forest of thirty-foot-high evergreens with grayish bark and dark green, glossy leaves with prominent seams. A breeze begins to rustle your hair, and a peppery fragrance fills the air that tickles your senses and lifts your spirits. You're approaching a plantation of allspice.

This aromatic member of the myrtle family was discovered by the Spaniards in the sixteenth century in Jamaica. It's native to the West Indies, the rain forests of Central and South America, and cultivated in Mexico and Honduras, but half of the world's supply comes from Jamaica. It is also known as *pimento*, *Jamaica pepper*, and *English spice*, because of its popularity in England.

At three years of age, the stately evergreens begin to bear fruit. Small white flowers bloom in June, July, and August, followed by rough, ribbed green berries that contain the vital pain-relieving eugenol, which is present in the rind of the berries *before* they ripen, but not after. To preserve this vital oil, the tiny, brittle berries of allspice are picked when they are fully grown but still green and unripe. They are sun-dried for days, until the berries become a burnished red-brown.

HEALTH VIRTUES: Allspice is a warming tonic with lots of zest and a flavor that herbalists often compare to cloves, juniper, cinnamon, and pepper. It's like getting four tastes in one spice. It's a carminative spice—one that is known for its ability to stimulate the production of digestive enzymes and ease digestive distress, including indigestion, gas, and bloating of the stomach. Its anesthetic oil, eugenol, eases muscle pain and tension in the gastrointestinal tract. It is also believed to have antioxidant properties. Since warming spices like allspice ease "cold" conditions, allspice has a history of use as a topical spice plaster for muscle pain, joint pain, and arthritis.

CULINARY PLEASURES: Allspice adds vigor to anything you sprinkle it on: meats, poultry, poached fish, stuffing, soups, stews, beans, and the heavier vegetables. It's also great with baked apples, pumpkin, and deviled eggs, or all alone in cottage cheese. In the Caribbean, allspice is a favorite for aromatic barbecue: allspice leaves are used in the stuffing for meats, and allspice wood is used as the fuel for a crackling, aromatic fire. It's popular in England for soups and stews, in Scandinavia for pickled herring, in the Middle East for meat and rice, and in India for curry.

USING ALLSPICE SEEDS: The dried seeds keep indefinitely, but you'll need a coffee grinder or food mill that doesn't have plastic parts to grind the seeds, because allspice seeds are hard. Powdered allspice provides greater ease and convenience, but it has a shorter shelf life than the whole dried seeds.

ANISE
Sweet Dreams

Pimpinella anisum
PART USED: Seeds, Pods

Sweet anise is one of the ancient herbs of the Mediterranean that was so revered, the Bible mentions it as an herb that was used to pay taxes. It happened again in England in the fourteenth century when the London Bridge was falling down, and King Edward I listed anise as a taxable herb. Anise can proudly say it helped to earn the fees to repair the London Bridge.

Aromatic anise is an annual member of the parsley family with long, smooth, pale green stems; thick, oval, bright green leaves at the base; and upper leaves that are feathery. It can grow one to two feet high, but because of its delicate nature, it tends to lie on the ground. In July and August, it blooms with tiny white flowers in starburst clusters, followed by brown fruits that contain anise's oil with the licorice flavor.

Anise is a native of the Mediterranean and Egypt, where it was used as a medicine and food in the sixteenth century. In ancient Greece and Rome, where feasting was king, anise was queen of the evening in cakes served at the end of the meal as digestive aids. The Roman armies brought anise to England, where it was used in pillows to prevent bad dreams. The linen of Edward IV of England was scented with anise for its sedative effect. You can sleep like royalty by tucking aniseed in your pillowcase.

HEALTH VIRTUES: Anise is a sweet-tasting herb with a warm, drying nature. It's anti-inflammatory, antifungal, and a pain reliever, with a long history of use as a digestive aid. It eases stomach discomfort, prevents fermentation in the intestines from undigested meats, and fights indigestion and gas. It was recommended by Hippocrates to treat respiratory conditions—it's an expectorant that breaks up congestion and mucus, good for stuffed-up sinuses, colds, coughs, and bronchitis, and good for people with asthma. Anise also has a history of use as a breath freshener. Anise honey is a time-honored tonic to fight emphysema. It's an herb to strengthen the liver, to fight hepatitis and cirrhosis, and it's believed to be helpful in warding off tumors.

CULINARY PLEASURES: Anise is a world favorite, and the whole plant is edible. The root can be eaten as a vegetable or used in salads and for sweetness in stir-fry dishes. The seeds add sweetness to soup, stew, cookies, cakes, candies, liquors, and wines—*anisette, absinthe, pernot, ouzo, muscatel.* Anise is often used as a substitute for licorice. Toss anise leaves or seeds into your salads to get the benefit of its vital health properties. Use anise in honey to power up your health and digestion.

USING ANISEED: Whole aniseed comes in shakers. The seeds are very small and brittle, and it's best to crush them with a pestle before using them. Once they are crushed, they lose their brittle nature in drinks or cooking.

BASIL
King of the Herbs

Ocimum basilicum

PART USED: Leaves, Flowers, Seeds

We will venture into a garden of love as we secretly follow a boy named Nicholas down a winding street in Italy. A dark-eyed girl approaches, and she blushes as she hands Nicholas a sprig of basil and runs off, giggling. Nicholas heaves a deep sigh and holds the aromatic sprig of basil close to his heart, because the girl he has been longing for has just given him a token of love from folklore that means, *Kiss me, Nicholas.*

This legendary member of the mint family is a native of India, Africa, and Asia. In India it is considered a sacred herb, protector of life and death, often placed in the hands of a loved one who has died to insure passage to paradise. Called king of the herbs, royal herb, and Saint Joseph's wort (plant), this treasured annual is often associated with divinity.

Sweet basil grows a square stem that branches prolifically, producing shiny oval leaves with serrated edges, in sweet and fragrant shades of greens and purples. From June to September, it blooms with small white or purple whorls of flowers.

Basil is cultivated around the world, particularly in the United States and Egypt. In ancient times, it was used as a charm against witchcraft and to invite prosperity and luck. In Romania, basil was given as a token to signify an engagement, and in Italy, it's all about love. A good friend's grandmother—Mom Mom Cilliberti from Calabria—recalled her youth in Italy when men used to put sprigs of basil behind their ears, like perfume.

HEALTH VIRTUES: The king of the herbs has a crowning list of health properties. It's an immune system stimulant that increases the production of antibodies to fight infections and disease. It's a circulatory stimulant that increases oxygen to the brain, and a *nervine*, an herb that strengthens the nervous system to fight all nervous disorders, including nervous tension headaches and depression. It's a blood builder and bacteria killer, including organisms that cause dysentery. It's an herb for recovery; with vitamins A and C and oil of camphor, it's an antiseptic for kidney cleansing and strengthens digestion. Basil has been used to restore strength in mothers after childbirth.

CULINARY PLEASURES: Fresh leaves are spicy; dried leaves are sweet. Use with anything that contains tomatoes: sauces, pizza, pesto, and green salads. It is often used in France's *bouquet garni* and in curry from Thailand. Basil is fabulous with light white fish, crabmeat, eggplant, and zucchini, and when sprinkled on cucumbers with Parmesan cheese.

BAY
The Daphne Tree

Laurus nobilis

PART USED: Leaves, Berries, Bark

Inhale the crisp fragrance of a bay leaf, and let yourself be transported back in time to the hills of ancient Greece, where you'll find a stately evergreen with a sheen on its smooth, gray bark and dramatically cut leaves that are thick, shiny, and dark green. You are in the presence of the Daphne tree, named for the maiden Daphne, who was transformed into a laurel to escape the passionate advances of Apollo.

The story begins with the notorious trickster Cupid, who was called to task by Apollo for his wanton mischief making in the name of love. Cupid's reaction wasn't what the sun god had expected—an apology. The trickster Cupid decided to show Apollo a thing or two about what love could do.

It was no secret on Olympus that Apollo had a wanton reputation of his own with innocent maidens he seduced at his whim. To pay Apollo back for chiding him, Cupid shot a golden arrow into Apollo to make him fall in love with the first woman he saw.

One morning, the maiden Daphne was taking a walk. Apollo saw her and was love struck. Cupid intervened and shot Daphne with an arrow of lead to harden her heart and make her repulsed by the first man she saw—Apollo. Daphne ran from Apollo, pleading for help, and the goddess Athena transformed Daphne into a laurel tree to preserve her innocence for eternity.

Heartsick with the loss of his love, Apollo picked the leaves from the laurel tree and made a crown of bay, which he wore from that day on to honor Daphne. Wreaths of bay replaced the standard wreaths of olive that crowned victors in the Olympic games in the eighth century in Greece, and later, the tradition was carried on in Rome to pay tribute to Apollo.

The laurel is considered a noble or holy tree in Greece. One legend claims that a bay tree can protect a person from lightning on the land where it is planted.

HEALTH VIRTUES: Herbs that have noble or religious associations also seem to have strong disease-fighting properties, and the leaves of the Daphne tree are blessed with healing virtues. Warm and drying, bay is a tonic for the nerves, sedating and relaxing. Its oil is antibacterial and antifungal to fight infections, particularly in the respiratory system. Used as a steam inhalant at the onset of a cold or flu, bay can kill the infection, clear the breathing passages, and remove congestion from the head and chest. It's also an herb for a healthy heart and arteries, to help to reduce blood pressure. Bay is an antidote for toxins, which makes it an excellent cleanser for the spleen, liver, glands, testicles, and joints—to fight rheumatism and arthritis, and to help to ward off tumors and cancer. Add bay to your menu if you suffer with headaches, nervous conditions, or nervous itching.

CULINARY PLEASURES: A treasured herb in France, bay is one of the herbs in *bouquet garni*. Bay is also popular in Italian, Spanish, Creole, and Indonesian cooking, for soup, stew, shellfish, sauces, marinades, poultry, and fish. It is used in gumbo, shrimp, and crab dishes in African American cuisine. A Balinese blend of aromatic leaves includes bay leaf, lemongrass, and pine leaves with rice, turmeric, and coconut milk—known as a sacred dish. Bay in beef dishes insures a richer flavor and a health-enriching gravy, and grandma's curative chicken soup isn't complete without bay.

USING BAY LEAVES: Remember to remove the bay leaves before serving the dish.

CARAWAY
Soothing Seeds

Carum carvi

PART USED: Seeds, Leaves, Root

The spicy fragrance of caraway seeds will take us back in time to colonial New England to see this ancient herb from Europe blooming in America for the first time in the gardens of the Pilgrims.

Colonial gardens in New England were plain and utilitarian, set near the house, with boundaries that were often defined by a square wooden fence. Here, vegetables and herbs were planted for daily food, including onions, leeks, garlic, radishes, carrots, cabbage, artichokes, and melons. Herbs were planted next to the vegetables in no particular arrangement—short next to tall, hardy next to delicate—giving the cook easy access to a standard meal, which was often a simmering meat stew with a variety of herbs and vegetables.

Aromatic herbs were planted in a separate area of the garden to prevent them from flavoring the soil where the vegetables grew. They were tied in bundles and hung in rooms as air fresheners, used in drawers with linens and as dyes for clothing, and often carried in the Pilgrims' pockets. The herbs that were used for medicines were dried and stored for use in the cold winters.

Roses were grown for their petals, which were used for fragrance, but if the lady of the house wanted flowers for her table, she would look to the land around her for inspiration, collecting mayflowers and violets from the fields and woods to transplant into her garden.

The intrinsic nature of a garden is to invite wild herbs in, while confined garden herbs spread their seeds on the wind. In this way, new herbs were propagated in lands where they had never been, while native herbs popped up in gardens unexpectedly, next to their herbal friends. In the early days of America, caraway was one of the herbs that escaped its confinement in colonial gardens and began to grow wild in North America. An herb that was as old as civilization, listed in the medical papyrus of Thebes from the sixteenth century, was loose in the winds of the New World.

Caraway is a biennial with branching stems, feathery leaves, and clusters of small, white flowers that bloom in midsummer, followed by long, brown, ribbed seeds. Dried seeds of this ancient herb were found among 5,000-year-old-remnants of the Swiss Lake Dwellers. Popular in European folklore, one legend claims that your valuable possessions can't be stolen if they contain caraway. It was used as an ingredient in love potions to keep lovers from straying. Farmers fed it to their chickens, geese, and pigeons to keep them loyal. Needless to say, there is something about caraway that keeps you coming back.

HEALTH VIRTUES: Caraway is a tonic for the stomach, to ease digestive upsets, gassy indigestion, and flatulence. It's antibacterial to fight infections, with a warming nature that relieves tension. Rich in hormones, it was used to regulate menses and ease cramps. Its vital properties are carvene and carvol (an oxygenated oil with menthol). The leaves contain the same properties as the seeds, and the roots are eaten as well, often compared to parsnips, but with a richer flavor. It's a gift in any garden—an herb that helps to strengthen memory and improve vision.

CULINARY PLEASURES: Caraway has been used in Germany for more than 1,000 years to season cabbage and reduce the acidic effects of sauerkraut. Caraway seeds are a flavoring in breads, especially rye. In Roman times, caraway roots were combined with milk to make caraway bread, a staple in the daily diet of Roman soldiers. There are caraway cookies, cakes, cheeses, and the German liquor called *kümmel*, which is used as a digestive aid. In medieval England, caraway was a popular companion for roasted apples, immortalized by Shakespeare in *Henry IV*, when Squire Shallow offered Falstaff "a pippin and a dish of caraway."

Dutch caraway seeds are considered the best for shape, color, and strength of their oil.

Egyptian caraway has a milder, less bitter flavor than Dutch caraway.

CARDAMOM
Grains of Paradise

Elettaria cardamomum

PART USED: Seeds

Before we begin our adventure, we will prepare a cup of coffee the Middle Eastern way, with crushed seeds of cardamom, steeped to heighten their flavor. As we sip this exotic treat with a floral, woody nature, a wind stirs the sands of time, and we find ourselves in 606 BC, in the Fertile Crescent of the Euphrates River, where the biblical city of Babylon was located. Nebuchadnezzar II has conquered the reigning Assyrian Empire, along with its capital city of Nineveh, called "the glory of kingdoms." With Nineveh's fall, the first Babylonian Empire ends, and the Neo-Babylonian Empire begins. It is here that one of the Seven Wonders of the Ancient World was created: the Hanging Gardens of Babylon.

Legend tells us that Nebuchadnezzar II had the gardens built as a tribute to his wife, Amyitis, to ease her depression at the loss of her homeland, the green and mountainous lands of Media (Persia), to the east of Babylon. She was the daughter of a prince of Media who had formed an alliance with Nebuchadnezzar to vanquish the Assyrians and restore the Babylonian Empire to its former glory as the first great kingdom of western Asia. Their conquest was so fierce and destructive that the ancient city of Ninevah was literally erased from the map. Nebuchadnezzar's kingdom spanned the deserts of southwestern Asia, with Babylon as his imperial city.

The riches from trade in the Mesopotamian kingdom would pass through the gates of Babylon. To secure his reign and project his image as the greatest ruler in the world, Nebuchadnezzar enslaved the skilled Assyrian craftsmen to rebuild Babylon on a grand scale. They began with the walls to fortify the city, and they were no ordinary walls.

The walls of Babylon were laid out in a square around the city, fifteen miles long on each side of the square, approximately seventy feet high, eighty-seven feet thick, and made of stone. Inside the walls of Babylon, extravagance reigned in the elaborate design of the royal palaces, luxurious temples to the Babylonian god, stately parks and hunting grounds, and the most remarkable feature of all, miles and miles of the Euphrates River running through the center of the city, sealed behind the walls.

Amid this grandeur, to the northeast of the royal palace, the Hanging Gardens of Babylon appeared like a botanical mirage, with vaulted terraces and arches, one on top of another in tiers that climbed as high as the city walls.

The terraces were connected by stairways that led to the upper balconies, and as guests climbed to the heights, above their heads they would see cascading trees, ferns, and exotic plants that were imported from around the world, glistening with moisture despite the Mesopotamian heat. The gardens must have seemed like a mirage suspended in the air.

Greek historian Diodorus Siculus wrote that the approach to the garden ". . . sloped like a hillside and the several parts of the structure rose from one another tier on tier . . . On all this, the earth had been piled and was thickly planted with trees of every kind. . . ."

The stone building that contained the hanging gardens was designed in a square a quarter mile long, supported by cube-shaped pillars that were hollowed out and filled with soil to serve as gigantic pots for larger trees—willow, cedar, cypress, olive, fruit, almond, date, palm, oak, fir, and myrtle, to name just a few.

Fountains within the gardens kept the foliage moist. The terraces were constructed from baked mud brick and bitumen, natural asphalt. This was insulated with watertight beams of palm tree trunks, mats of reeds, and layers of lead to keep the water from leaking into the chambers below. It was a masterwork of architecture and technology that defied the imagination—a mountain of greenery thriving on brick terraces in a scorched desert environment. The gardens were fed from the Euphrates River with hydraulic pumps that sent water to reservoirs at heights never dreamed. The pumps were manned by slaves, working in shifts to turn a screw that has been compared to an Archimedes' screw.

Diodorus Siculus wrote, ". . . the water machines [raised] the water in great abundance from the river, though no one outside could see it being done."

In this lofty garden, we are looking for the aromatic seeds of cardamom, but we will have to come down from the heights. It's a spice that was known to rich and poor alike. There was an old saying in the Middle East, "A poor man would rather give up his bread than his daily cardamom," and for a good reason. Cardamom cools the body, which is a blessing under the sun, in Mesopotamian heat.

Cardamom is a large bush that can reach sixteen feet in height, with dark green leaves that can be as long as two feet and as wide as six inches. On the base of the bush, leafy stalks snake along the ground. They bloom with green flowers that have white tips with purple veins, followed by rough seedpods. Inside the pods, small, sticky seeds are lined up in double rows, six seeds to a row, with a deep brown-black color.

This native of India is the second most expensive spice in the world (saffron is first). It was known as an aphrodisiac by the ancient Arab traders, chewed in ancient Egypt as a breath freshener and cleanser for the teeth, and used by the Vikings 1,000 years ago. It is cultivated in Sri Lanka, Indochina, Tanzania, and Guatemala.

HEALTH VIRTUES: Cardamom is a pungent spice with a warming nature and undertones of lemon. It has a long history of use as a medicine and food, and a reputation for being the best aphrodisiac. It's a carminative spice, one that stimulates the production of digestive enzymes to ease bloating and gas. It was used by the Romans to combat the distress that accompanied late-night feasting. It's also calming for the central nervous system, and it moves chi (vital energy). According to Chinese medicine, stagnant chi leads to nervous conditions, headaches, irritability, and a host of nervous disorders.

CULINARY PLEASURES: Cardamom is an ingredient in curry, Middle Eastern coffee, and a popular spice in cuisine of the Far East. The seeds are used in Scandinavian baked breads and apple pie, Dutch windmill biscuits, pickles, pickled herring, and mulled wine. Cardamom brings an exotic flavor to beef, chicken, and sweet potatoes.

USING CARDAMOM SEEDS: The whole seeds (inside the pod) have the richest taste and aroma, and black cardamom is the most potent. To use whole seeds, break open the outer pod, which is tasteless, remove the dark brown seeds inside, and grind them with a mortar and pestle. An alternative method is to bruise the seeds and fry them before combining them with other ingredients. You can buy the pods split or whole, and the seeds are also sold loose. Once cardamom seeds are ground, they quickly lose their flavor and aroma, so it's best to use them just as the dish comes off the heat. Preground cardamom seeds are available, which provide greater convenience in exchange for less potency and aroma.

CAYENNE
Red-Hot Momma of Healers

Capsicum frutescens

PART USED: Fruit, Leaves

We will have to peruse a garden of synonyms to get this pepper straight. Called American red pepper, African red pepper, Spanish pepper, red pepper, capsicum, cayenne, chile, chile pepper, garden pepper, even bird pepper, cayenne was used as a medicinal spice for centuries, in a class by itself. Other peppers can be irritating, but cayenne is not. It is known for its soothing nature and healing virtues.

HEALTH VIRTUES: Cayenne is regarded as a panacea with health properties that work on many fronts. It's a stimulant and body tonic for conditions that have a "cold nature," such as exhaustion, chronic fatigue, and shock from a fall, injury, or loss. It's a powerful infection fighter, with antiseptic, antifungal, and antibacterial properties. It contains a top-notch pain reliever—capsicin/capsaicin—for deep muscle pain, back pain, deep nerve pain, sprains, arthritis, rheumatism, fibromyalgia, and shingles. It stimulates circulation to bring oxygen to the brain for better concentration and memory. It stimulates the production of saliva and digestive enzymes to strengthen digestion. A spice for a healthy heart, it helps to strengthen arteries, capillaries, and veins. It increases sweating to eliminate toxins from the body, and reduces fevers, inflammation, and swelling in glands and joints. It's a spice for cold hands and feet and circulatory problems related to diabetes. Cayenne also strengthens the intestines, protects the stomach lining, helps to regulate blood sugar, and helps to burn fat. It is rich in nutrients, including vitamins A, C (bioflavonoids), and B-complex, and zinc, iron, calcium, potassium, magnesium, phosphorus, sulfur, sodium, selenium, and pectin.

CULINARY PLEASURES: Cayenne is a world favorite spice for pepper lovers. Use it sparingly, since a little will go a long way. If you find it too hot straight, try chile powder, a blend of cayenne and milder peppers. That way, you can get the benefits of cayenne without the hot taste.

NOTE: Wash your hands after touching cayenne so you don't get it in your eyes. If you get it in your eyes, you'll feel a hot sensation, but don't panic. Wash your eyes thoroughly with water, and if they still bother you, follow with eye drops. Avoid cayenne if you have weak kidneys. It's not for children.

CELERY
Cleansing Seeds

Apium graveolens

PART USED: Seeds, Root, Stems

We'll take a morning walk along the coast of Wales to look for a member of the carrot family and kin of parsley, growing wild. It's a bright green herb that can reach two to three feet in height, with thick, shiny stems and glossy leaves with ruffled edges. It flowers with small white blossoms in clusters, and on closer inspection, we can see that the stems have many fine ridges and the herb has a grassy fragrance that is enchanting.

The wild variety of celery is far more fragrant than the celery we know as a vegetable, and it was believed to be an aphrodisiac in ancient Greece and Rome. Known for more than 3,000 years, celery was used as a medicine and food in ancient Egypt and in China in the fifth century BC. Celery was known as *smallage* in the Middle Ages, a wild marsh plant in coastal soils like England and Wales. Italian farmers began to cultivate smallage for food, and over the years, celery lost the bitter aspect it had in the wilds, and its fragrance became weaker, but the taste and texture improved. The stems are used as vegetables around the world, but the vital properties are weaker in the stems. The power is in the seeds.

HEALTH VIRTUES: A rich, volatile oil is present in celery seeds. One of its characteristics is to calm the central nervous system with a gentle, tranquilizing effect—to ease tension, anxiety, nervous disorders, and digestive stress. Celery seeds are also a natural antacid and antiseptic to cleanse the bladder and fight urinary tract infections. They remove uric acid from kidneys and stimulate blood flow, which flushes wastes from the muscles and joints—beneficial for arthritis. Chinese studies show that celery lowers blood pressure. The seeds are rich in potassium, sodium, calcium, iron, silicon, and vitamins A, B-complex, and C.

CULINARY PLEASURES: Celery is a good seasoning for people who can't eat onions or are on a low-salt diet. The seeds add a crunchy flavor to many dishes, including creamed chicken and turkey, cream cheese, dips, tomato juice, stewed tomatoes, eggs, meat loaf, hamburgers, stew, soup, chowder, fish, salad dressing, coleslaw, potato salad, fruit salad, sandwich spreads, vegetables, relishes, and pickles.

CHERVIL
Herb of Joy

Anthriscus cerefolium

PART USED: Leaves, Root

To capture the essence of chervil, we will visit a very special cooking school in the 1950s in Paris, France. It was located in a rooftop kitchen on the rue de L'Universite—the first school run by Julia Child. Here she taught the intricate subtleties that define the art of French cuisine: how to get maximum puff from egg whites, how to stuff a cabbage leaf by leaf, how to flip a sizzling omelet with a flick of the wrist. As the world came to know and love her from her books and TV, we discovered that the art of individuality was one of her greatest gifts. She was a fountain of joy, spontaneity, and wry humor. She showed us how to be nonchalant when the towel catches fire or the chicken hits the floor, and how to have fun with just about anything.

Once she spent two years and 284 pounds of flour to master the art of French bread. With all of her brilliance, attention to detail, and patience for experimentation that inspired awe, she had a way of sifting complexities down to sheer delight. For example, she wrapped up the intricate and detailed introduction to volume 2 of *Mastering the Art of French Cooking* by calling it "this leisurely meander."

She had a light in her eyes, like a divine spark, and it lingers still. She reminds us to keep our knives sharp, and above all, "have a good time."

In France, chervil is used like parsley, often called French parsley. This aromatic member of the carrot family has a sweet flavor and an uplifting nature. Its Latin name means *herb of joy*. It's a beautiful plant that loves hills and pastures, thrives in wet places, prefers slanted light and shade, and tends to hug hedges. Its leaves are remarkable—finely cut and lacy green. Chervil flowers in clusters of delicate white blossoms.

Chervil was used as a potherb by the Romans and cultivated in Brazil as early as the seventeenth century. There are so many species of chervil all of them have yet to be identified, but the last count named more than forty. The chervil we know as the official herb with a hint of anise is garden chervil that is native to eastern Europe and western Asia. The Romans brought chervil to France, where it inspired such delight, it became one of the herbs used in the fines herbes blend.

HEALTH VIRTUES: Chervil is a spirit-lifting herb that warms the stomach and eases digestion. It's a fine herb to use for any "cold" condition. It helps to lower blood pressure and maintain a healthy respiratory system, since it is an expectorant for phlegm. It has a long history of use as a treatment for anemia and menses disorders.

CULINARY PLEASURES: Chervil's best use is in a blend with other herbs. It's popular in Europe for soups, spice blends, poultry, fish, and vegetables, and as a complement to vinegar. It's an ingredient in German green sauce. The most delightful way to use chervil is fresh, and fresh leaves can be frozen to preserve their flavor. Dried chervil is not as aromatic as the fresh herb, but many cooks delight in the dried variety. In fact, dried chervil is one of the ingredients in the French blend for herbes de Provence.

CHILE POWDER
A blend of peppers and herbs that will vary, but will contain cayenne (chile pepper, red pepper) and often paprika, parsley, and resins of carrot as binders. Be sure to check the ingredients on the shaker of chile powder before you buy it to insure that you are getting only the peppers, herbs, and natural binders. You don't want MSG, sugar, or artificial coloring or flavoring, and I found several blends that had them.

CHIVES
The Health Builder

Allium schoenoprasum

PART USED: Leaves, Flowers, Bulbs

We will visit an herbal window garden in a Norwegian kitchen to find this spunky member of the lily family with its cascade of lean, green leaves that shoot up like reeds, straight from the bulb. It flowers in summer with decorative blossoms in pale purple or white puffs that look like fluffy balls.

Our hostess invites us to stay for scrambled eggs. She clips fresh, young shoots of chives from her window garden to garnish the eggs as they come off the heat. She tells us that an herbal window garden without chives wouldn't be Norwegian, and scrambled eggs without chives would be unthinkable. The winters are cold in Norway, but chives still thrive in indoor kitchen gardens, where they are often planted in a box, along with parsley, as snipping favorites.

Chives have two close cousins, onions and leeks, which also grow from bulbs. In Germany chives are called *cuttable leeks*. Chives' Latin name—*Allium*—means *garlic*, and the lean, green leaves have a mild garlic flavor.

In the Middle Ages, when illness and disease were believed to be caused by evil spirits, chives were one of the herbs that were used to drive evil spirits away. Chives are native to China, where the stems are denser than other varieties; they are also native to Taiwan, and cultivated in California.

HEALTH VIRTUES: Chives are antibacterial to fight infections and boost your healing power. They contain chlorophyll, an oxygenator for cells and tissues to keep them healthy. They are also a blood builder with a healthy supply of strengthening nutrients, including sulfur for healthy hair, skin, pituitary, pancreas, nerves, metabolism, cell building, and removal of toxins. Chives have a warm, drying nature to counter the effects of cold, damp conditions such as rheumatism and colds with mucous conditions. They also promote good digestion, help to lower blood pressure and cholesterol, are cleansing for the liver, and help to digest fats. Chives are an excellent source of vitamin C (an antioxidant), folic acid, calcium (for strong bones and prevention of intestinal polyps), iron, and potassium.

CULINARY PLEASURES: Chives have a tangy flavor that flatters scrambled eggs, deviled eggs, egg salads, beans, cream soups, and corn and fish chowders. The minced bulb is often fried with bacon bits as a topping for baked potatoes. In cream cheese and cottage cheese, chives are a standard. You can get a healthy supply of chives in your menu by routinely tossing them into your green salads. When you use chives in cooked dishes, add them at the end to preserve the vitamin C.

USING FRESH CHIVES: If you use chives fresh from your window garden, the young, tender leaves are recommended for culinary use. After the plant flowers, the stems are tough; therefore, it's best to keep chives cut back to discourage blooming, in order to have a ready supply of young, tender reeds, which will be generated quickly as you snip. You can grow a second plant in your window garden to use strictly for chive flowers, which have the same properties as the leaves and add color and energy to any salad. Fresh chives have a mellow flavor, while dried chives are more tart.

CILANTRO The fresh leaves and stems of the coriander plant. See Coriander.

CINNAMON
Earthy Treasure

Cinnamomum burmanni, cassia

PART USED: Inner Bark

As we inhale the sweet, woody fragrance of cinnamon, the spice with a warming nature, we travel back in time to visit the tropical forest of Sri Lanka, the home of true cinnamon in the wilds. We are looking for an evergreen that loves high altitudes and lots of rain. The tree can reach a height of sixty feet in the wilds, but the average is twenty to thirty feet; it has a soft, reddish brown bark, shiny green leathery leaves, and white blossoms.

The burnished brown sticks of cinnamon are called *quills*. They come from the inner bark of young trees that are propagated by cuttings from the larger trees. This protects the larger trees from extinction, which sadly happened in the rain forests of South America, when wild trees were used as a source for the spice. During the rainy season, the young trees are cut back, and the bark is removed and left to ferment for at least one day. When the outer bark is fermented, it is scraped off, exposing the inner bark, which is dried in the sun. Exposure to the sun causes the inner bark to curl into quills (rolled sticks) that are a sweet reddish brown.

Cinnamon is a spice that has been adored around the world since the dawn of time. It was one of the most popular spices in the cache of the Arab traders, who told wild tales about the origin of cinnamon being a mountain range in Arabia where birds of prey used cinnamon to make their nests. It was one of the first spices sought in European explorations for its sweet, pungent taste and earthy fragrance. The discovery of America is often credited to cinnamon, since Christopher Columbus was looking for the Spice Islands, where cinnamon grew, but he veered off course and found America.

Cinnamon was mentioned in the Torah and has a long history of use in India and Egypt dating back to 500 BC. It is native to India, China, and Japan, and cultivated in tropical climates around the world, including the Philippines and West Indies.

HEALTH VIRTUES: Cinnamon is an antiseptic spice that fights bacterial, fungal, viral, and yeast infections, including E. coli and candida. It's a cleansing spice for the sinuses and mucous conditions. It stimulates circulation, which helps to maintain a healthy body, brain, and heart, and it helps to reduce high blood pressure. Current studies show that cinnamon reduces blood sugar levels to fight adult-onset diabetes. It is also a digestive aid to ease indigestion and gas. It has a history of use as a medicine in China and Japan where it is a native (*Cinnamomum cassia*). It has also been used to treat menses and uterine difficulties.

CULINARY PLEASURES: Used in Asian spice blends for many dishes, in fruit filling, and apple and peach pandowdy in African American cuisine. Commonly known as a spice for breads, fruits, cereals, muffins, cakes, cookies, and exotic spice blends.

Sri Lanka cinnamon is *Cinnamomum zeylanicum*, known as *true* cinnamon. Traditionally, the inner bark of wild trees was used to provide the spice.

Indonesian cinnamon is *Cinnamomum burmanni*—commonly used in the United States.

Vietnamese cinnamon (called Saigon cinnamon) is *Cinnamomum loureirii*, often called the *best* cinnamon.

CLOVE
Buds of Plenty

Eugenia caryophyllata, Syzygium aromaticum
PART USED: Dried Flower Buds

For this herbal adventure, we will pack a straw hat and an airtight jar for dried flower buds that we'll collect as we go island hopping. Our first getaway will take us to the evergreen forests in the Mollucan islands of Indonesia, and to the Philippines, where this member of the myrtle family is a native. We are looking for a pyramid-shaped tree with a bounty of rich green tapered leaves that have deep center spines, and we will have to look up, since the clove tree can grow to a height of fifty feet.

Our next stop for flower buds will be the islands where the clove tree is widely cultivated: Madagascar and Tanzania, where luck is with us, because pink buds are just beginning to appear on the clove trees, and it's an opportunity to see the buds before they are picked—new and unopened. We complete our bud collection in the West Indies and finally Brazil, where we will relax in an open-air café, lay our buds on the table, and watch how people waft into our vicinity, enchanted by the aromatic fragrance of the spice from the pyramid trees.

Cloves were an early favorite in the spice trade, arriving in Alexandria, Egypt, in 176 AD. The unopened flower buds are pink when they are picked and dry to a deep, rich brown under the sun. They were used as a cure-all in southeast Asia for thousands of years. In the Mollucan islands, cloves were inserted into oranges to use as an insect repellent, a helpful hint to chase insects from our yards with a natural insecticide.

HEALTH VIRTUES: The volatile oil of cloves consists of four oils that are antibacterial, antiseptic, and antiparasitic to ward off infections (viral, bacterial, and fungal), and to expel parasites. It contains a potent anti-inflammatory and anesthetic for pain relief, eugenol, which can be 60–80 percent of the oil of cloves. It is soothing to the gastrointestinal tract to fight indigestion, bloating, and gas; and cleansing and strengthening for the stomach, liver, spleen, and skin. It fights toxins and can help to ward off tumors. It's also a stimulant for the body and mind and an aphrodisiac. It contains a natural aspirin compound and the antioxidant vanillin, and is a good source of vitamin C, omega-3 fatty acids, calcium, magnesium, manganese, and fiber.

CULINARY PLEASURES: Cloves are a popular ingredient in spice blends from India, Asia, and the Middle East, including the potent Chinese five-spice powder, and a main ingredient in clove lemonade in African American cuisine. Cloves give ketchup its zip; they are used in Germany for cookies, and cloves are a standard for meat dishes, pickles, salad dressings, and Worcestershire sauce blends.

CORIANDER
Manna from Heaven

Coriandrum sativum

PART USED: Seeds, Leaves

What garden can we visit to capture the essence of this slender, ancient herb from the parsley family that is renowned for its seeds? The timeless garden of Exodus 16:31, where coriander was compared to the manna from heaven, which were seeds for bread that fell from the sky to feed the Israelites in exile.

"And the house of Israel called the name thereof Manna: and it was like coriander seed, white; and the taste was like wafers made with honey."

We are looking for a native plant of the Middle East that stands about two feet tall on a round stem. Its bright green, shiny leaves have two distinct leaf patterns: oval and divided at the base or linear and feathery on the top. Small flowers bloom in umbels (like spokes in an umbrella, attached to a single stem). The flowers are delicate and white, with the palest hint of mauve. The seeds are tiny and round, also clustered, and they fall from the plant when they are ripe.

The leaves and unripe seeds of coriander will give off a strange odor as we approach, and for this reason, it repels all insects, but as the seeds ripen, they become sweet and fragrant and have been used as an aphrodisiac for centuries. In the Arabian classic, *One Thousand and One Nights*, a tale is told of a merchant who was still childless in his forties, until he took a potion that contained coriander.

Stories of coriander date back thousands of years. In Egypt, where it grows wild, it is used as a medicine and food. It is also known as Chinese parsley, and in China, it is viewed as an herb that grants immortality. Coriander was mentioned in Sanskrit texts from India, and dried seeds of coriander were discovered in the ruins of the shops at Pompeii, when the city was excavated. It was known to Hipppocrates and Pliny, and it grew in the gardens of Charlemagne, the emperor of the Roman Empire in the first century AD. It was brought to England by the Romans, introduced to Mexico by Spanish conquistadores, and was one of the herbs in gardens of the American colonists, where it became a runaway, growing wild in North America.

HEALTH VIRTUES: Coriander is a stimulating spice that is antibacterial and antifungal, with a long history of use as a digestive aid. It increases the production of gastric juices to improve digestion and tone the stomach, which increases the vitality of every body system. It is also a spice for the heart, to lower cholesterol, and it helps to reduce blood sugar levels to fight diabetes. Its soothing nature is calming for the central nervous system, to ease tension and stress, and the aches of arthritis and rheumatism. It has been used to ease the pains of childbirth.

CULINARY PLEASURES: In the case of coriander, only the seeds and root are known as coriander, while the leaves are known as cilantro.

The whole plant and the root are used, but the seeds have the richest flavor.

Leaves—Cilantro: The leaves are used like parsley but often in denser amounts. Egyptians and Peruvians use coriander leaves in soups. It's a favored herb in Asian, Mexican, South American, Spanish, and Caribbean cuisine. In the southwestern United States, cilantro is a standard in salads, burritos, salsa, and meats. In the Middle East, the leaves are used in chutney and curry. The leaves lose their flavor when they are dried, but you can freeze chopped cilantro in ice cube trays. *Note:* I've heard many people say they aren't fond of the taste of cilantro. If you agree, don't dismiss coriander from your menu. Try the seeds in rice or meat, and you'll change your mind.

Seeds—Coriander: The seeds are used in curry powder, stew, soup, rice, meats, breads, cakes, and sweets, including English black pudding. Popular in Arab dishes with lamb, combined with cumin in falafel, in Middle Eastern coffee, and north African red pepper sauce called *harissa*. Coriander combines well with cottage cheese and cream and is used to flavor liquors that are digestive aids. The seeds are nectar when they are mixed with honey—like manna from heaven.

USING CORIANDER SEEDS: The whole seeds have a long shelf life and become more fragrant as they age. To experience the richest flavor of coriander, use whole seeds, which you can easily grind with a mortar and pestle, since the seeds are brittle. If you buy the shaker variety in a see-through bottle, switch the contents to an airtight, dark bottle to preserve the spice longer. Even though powdered coriander seed in a shaker doesn't have the long shelf life of whole seeds, it's still aromatic, with an undertone of citrus that is deep and rich. (See chapter 22, "Magic Teaspoon Iced Teas," to find coriander in a fabulous iced tea.)

CUMIN
The Comforter

Cuminum cyminum
PART USED: **Seeds**

The warm, musty fragrance of this ancient spice takes us to the deserts of ancient Egypt, cumin's native home. Here we will find dried seeds of cumin in the highest place of honor, the pyramids of the Old Kingdom.

This member of the parsley family is a gentle, drooping plant, just under a foot tall, with slender, spear-shaped green leaves that have a tint of blue. It blossoms in June and July with clusters of small pink or white flowers. The seeds are hairy, brown, and boat-shaped, with bristly, tapered tips. Nine ridges run lengthwise along the seeds. The ancient Greeks for some reason associated cumin with greed, and the secret name for their emperor, Marcus Aurelius, was Cuminus. In Greece and Rome it was used as a medicine and in cosmetics to whiten the complexion. It is cultivated in India, China, and north Africa.

HEALTH VIRTUES: Cumin has a long history of use as a medicine in the East to the current day. It's a soothing spice for gastric distress, including dyspepsia, and for easing digestion and reducing bloating and gas. It's relaxing to the muscles, to reduce spasms and tension. It has been used to reduce nausea in pregnancy and to regulate menses. It is also used topically (in a poultice) to reduce swelling in the testicles and breasts, and for warts and tumors.

CULINARY PLEASURES: Cumin's deep, nutty flavor is often used in combination with other spices in blends. It is a major ingredient in curry and chile powders of India and spice blends in Syria, Iran, Pakistan, and Turkey. It is a popular spice in Morocco, Thailand, Vietnam, India, Spain, and Portugal. An ingredient in Mexican chili con carne and enchiladas with chile sauce. It's found in Middle Eastern couscous, stews and fish dishes, and in black beans and Creole rice in

African American cuisine. It is used in chutneys, sausages, and spiced cheeses—Munster from Germany and Leyden from the Netherlands. A popular drink in India, zeera pani, is made with tamarind water and cumin. It is also a spice for lamb, chicken, meat stews, and rice and bean dishes.

USING CUMIN SEEDS: The seeds need heat to release their potent aroma. Cooked dishes will accomplish this, but it's best to lightly roast or panfry whole or ground seeds before use in cold sauces and dishes. To season like a Mexican chef, vigorously rub the seeds between your palms to bruise them and let them fall into the dish while it is cooking. Use a light hand to avoid overpowering a dish; a half teaspoon is sufficient for a dish for two. Store ground cumin in an airtight container in a cool place to preserve its flavor.

DILL
Lullabye for the Nerves

Anethum graveolens

PART USED: Seeds, Oil, Leaves

As we inhale the sweet green fragrance of this dark green, feathery herb, we can travel in time to Europe in the 800s, when Charlemagne—Charles the Great, king of the Franks—was crowned Roman emperor. During his reign, Charlemagne issued a series of imperial edicts called capitularies (chapters), which delineated the royal position on civil, military, and religious affairs. One edict in particular—*the Capitulare de villis*—was one of the most remarkable documents ever issued by a king. It listed the names of specific plants that would be grown on royal estates and by association in the gardens of nobles and commoners alike. Ornamental flowers had been popular in gardens, but only two plants in Charlamagne's list were considered ornamental—the rose and the lily—and the rest were herbs. The list included anise, bay, caraway, celery, chervil, chives, coriander, cumin, fennel, garlic, mint, mustard, onion, parsley, poppy, rosemary, sage, and savory, to name just a few, and one of Charlemagne's favorite herbs, feathery dill.

Charlemagne was familiar with the health virtues of dill as a digestive aid, and one of his requirements for royal banquet tables was a crystal vial of dill for his guests, who were known to feast with such abandon, they often got hiccups.

HEALTH VIRTUES: Dill comes from the Old Norse *dilla*, which means to lull, and lull it does, in addition to curing hiccups. Dill is an aromatic nerve tonic, one of the most soothing herbs in the herbal kingdom to calm the entire body and steady the nerves. Dill in the system is like a sigh of relief. It eases stress, tension, digestive distress, and the jitters. Any disorder related to nerves is dill's territory, including a restless mind state and the inability to get to sleep. Dill fights infections, reduces swelling and pain, stimulates respiration for better breathing, calms a rapid heart rate, and dilates the blood vessels, which helps to reduce high blood pressure. It has a tradition of use for treating jaundice, E. coli, uterine problems, and fibroids. Dill is rich in minerals, including vitamin C (flavonoids), and very high in calcium, which helps to prevent intestinal polyps while it builds strong bones.

CULINARY PLEASURES: Well known in pickles, dill is also a favorite for shellfish and seafood, meats, cream cheese, cottage cheese, salad dressings, and dips. Dill is a popular seasoning in the Middle East for vegetables and rice pilaf, and a seasoning for Greek grape leaves. See chapter 8 for Dill Deliverance puree to get all of the benefits of dill, along with a blood builder.

FENNEL
Titan of Health

Foeniculum vulgare

PART USED: Seeds

We'll pay another visit to the garden of Greek lore to find the Titan Prometheus picking a stalk of fennel for a mission he has in mind. It was an ancient way to carry fire—in the hollow stalk of fennel. Prometheus is a giant, the son of the earth mother Gaea, and it is his responsibility to look after mortals, which legend says he fashioned out of clay. Caring for mortals is no easy task, since the god Zeus is out to get mortals at every bend in the road. Up to this point, Prometheus—whose name means *forethought*—has always been able to think of a way to outsmart Zeus for special compensations for the mortals in his keep. But this time, Zeus has gone too far. He has taken one of the essential elements of life away from mortals: fire.

Prometheus realizes that he has no tricks he can use to outsmart Zeus for fire, and his mortals will be doomed without it. There is no other choice; he must get fire and risk the temper of Zeus to do it. He takes the stalk of fennel to Olympus (heaven), hides fire from the sun in its stalk, and brings it to his earthbound friends.

He pays a price. Tied to a rock, Prometheus has to endure sacrificing his liver every day to a pecking bird, only to find his liver being restored every night. It's interesting to note one of the subtleties in this myth. The liver is the only organ in the human body that can regenerate itself, even if a section is removed. Perhaps our livers owe their regenerating nature to Prometheus's titan endurance, since he wasn't freed from the rock for 30,000 years. The other gift he gave us was the ability to cook food. If honors should go where honors are due, a fennel wreath should be placed on Prometheus's head to crown him father of the culinary arts.

Fennel is a tall and statuesque member of the carrot family with a glossy sheen on its stems and feathery leaves. Its small yellow flowers bloom in clusters, followed by small, brown, oval seeds with a hint of green and a licorice fragrance. When the seeds harden, they are harvested.

HEALTH VIRTUES: A titan herb for health, fennel is a natural anti-inflammatory and a circulatory tonic with a generous supply of nutrients for vigor and strength. It contains essential fatty acids and flavenoids, including rutin, vitamins A, C, and E, zinc, calcium, magnesium, phosphorus, sulfur, sodium, silica, iron, manganese, and selenium. Fennel is a natural antacid and well-respected herb for digestive disorders, including heartburn, acidity, constipation, and stomach discomfort. It helps to stimulate the production of digestive enzymes, and it has a calming effect on the entire digestive tract. It's also a natural diuretic that eases bloating, swelling in the hands, legs, and ankles, and hormonal puffiness. Romans believed that snakes got their powerful vision from the juice of fennel, since they were always rubbing against the plant for its juice.

Fennel tea is a time-honored treatment for weight control, since excess weight is closely related to digestive disturbances. It is also a natural antiseptic to flush wastes and toxins from the urinary tract. In Chinese medicine, fennel is used to tone the kidneys and spleen and treat urinary tract disorders and abdominal stress. It was one of the herbs used by Greek marathon runners. Known to Pilgrims as meeting seed, fennel was chewed during church services to calm the stomach and keep hunger pangs at bay.

CULINARY PLEASURES: Fennel is one of the herbs used in curry, Chinese five-spice powder, and herbes de Provence in France. Popular in Italy, Scandinavia, and China, fennel is used to flavor sausages, fish, and cakes, as well as liquors that are digestive aids. See chapter 22 to find fennel in Green Tea Sunrise, an invigorating iced tea.

GARLIC
Heal-All

Allium sativum

PART USED: Cloves

We will visit the land of the pharaohs, but we won't venture into the gilded palaces or hidden tombs. We're interested in the communities that were built near the pyramids for the pyramid builders, since we are curious about their menus. These were men who had to have Herculean energy and had to be fed well to insure their survival. Laboring in the sun hoisting stones to staggering heights was a job that required stamina and resistance to diseases in a climate that was all heat, a breeding ground for bacteria. Two herbs were prominent features in the diets of the pyramid builders: one was onion, and the other was garlic—known as heal-all—a supreme herb for healing. It was used in Egypt 4,000 years ago for strength and endurance, heart problems, respiratory problems, and tumors.

This perennial member of the lily family grows straight up from a bulb, two to three feet tall. It has a thick stem, a sparse selection of bright green, spear-shaped leaves, and blossoms that can be pale pink or white with a tint of green.

One of the most ancient herbs, garlic was used in the Middle East 5,000 years ago. It was also an herb of the Vikings—men who were legendary for their strength and endurance. It was used by Hippocrates and taken as a stimulant by Greek athletes before competitions. In Russia it is known as Russian penicillin.

HEALTH VIRTUES: Garlic contains a natural antibiotic with the strength of penicillin and no side effects. It's the herb to use for infections. It's anticancer, antiaging, antiviral, antifungal, antibacterial, and antiseptic. It's an immune system stimulant and a free radical scavenger, and it kills parasites. Garlic has a long history of use for all infections, including staph, strep, tuberculosis, polio, and plagues. It has been extensively researched in Japan, Germany, and the United States. It is good for the glands, including the lymph glands and thyroid. Garlic increases the production of interferon in the body, which helps to fight cancer. It contains selenium and germanium, which are also anticancer. It also helps to reduce blood sugar levels. A heart tonic with an anticlotting agent, it helps to lower cholesterol and blood pressure and reduce hypertension. Garlic contains enzymes that protect the liver from toxins, including lead.

Garlic contains a pyramid of health virtues: one-fourth sulfur (a health protector) as well as phosphorus, potassium, manganese, zinc, calcium, magnesium, sodium, iron, copper, vitamins A, B-complex, and C, and amino acid proteins. Garlic increases metabolic heat, which helps to burn fat. It provides energy during dieting, to fight fatigue. It is used for middle-ear infections and to tighten loose teeth. It's also an expectorant. I've heard many people say that they don't eat garlic because they don't want garlic breath. No problem: to counter garlic breath, chew parsley and add parsley to dishes that contain garlic. When you cook with garlic, the flavor mellows, and garlic breath isn't an issue.

CULINARY PLEASURES: An herb in every cuisine, garlic is used with eggs, meat, fish, poultry, potatoes, rice, beans, and vegetables, and in soup, sauces, dips, spice blends, and salads.

GINGER
Warmth

Zingiber officinale
PART USED: **Root**

The garden for this warm and fragrant golden spice would have to be the garden that lives in the ancient memory of every spiritual person. This golden root was so adored in Europe, it was believed to be an herb from the Garden of Eden.

Ginger is a perennial herb known for the gold in its rhizome (root fingers). The plant can grow to three feet in height, with lance-shaped leaves and stalks of small white or yellow flowers. When the herb is approximately ten months old, the rhizome is removed from the earth, washed, and soaked (and sometimes boiled) for cooking and sale.

From Africa, Asia, and Jamaica, ginger is cultivated in tropical climates around the world, including China and India

Ginger is the spice that gave birth to ginger ale, when it was added as a spice to beer and ale.

HEALTH VIRTUES: Ginger is a world-renowned medicinal herb with a warm, soothing nature. It is anti-inflammatory, antiviral, antiseptic, and an antitoxin, with anticancer properties. It's a well-respected circulatory tonic, lowers cholesterol, reduces high blood pressure, is anticlotting, and helps to reduce risk of heart attacks and strokes. Ginger is known for its ability to treat motion sickness, morning sickness, vertigo, and nausea, including that caused by chemotherapy and postoperative nausea. It has a long tradition of use for digestive disorders; it stimulates saliva and digestive enzymes and eases pain and discomfort in the stomach. Warming and comforting for coughs, colds, flu, and respiratory infections, ginger is an herb for healthy glands, kidneys, and bladder, because of its ability to remove wastes and toxins. It is soothing for rheumatoid arthritis, osteoarthritis, gout, and rheumatism. It's an important herb for recovery from illness, it's an energizer, and it helps to burn fat.

CULINARY PLEASURES: Ginger's pungent, lemony flavor is found in many cuisines: Asian, Indian, African American, Greek, and Egyptian. It blends well with everything from soup to nuts. Crystallized ginger comes from Australia.

HORSERADISH

Armoracia rusticana

PART USED: Root

The easiest way to use horseradish is from a prepared blend. Horseradish is one of the mustard herbs with stimulating properties. It's a digestive aid and one of the best herbs for water retention and edema. Horseradish also helps to strengthen blood vessels and lower high blood pressure. It fosters healthy kidneys and pancreas, acts as a natural laxative, and has a long history of use for respiratory congestion and as a poultice for muscle aches and pains from gout and arthritis. Horseradish is also rich in vitamin C and has antiseptic properties to fight flu, fevers, and infections.

LAVENDER
Herb of Harmony

Lavandula officinalis

PART USED: Flowers

We might take a day off to get lost in lavender, since there are twenty-eight species that vary in the cut and color of the leaves, with blossoms that range in color from white to lavender blue, which has a deep purple tint. Wherever there is lavender, there is an intoxicating fragrance in the air. We'll find it in vases on café tables in southern France, where lavender is used in herbes de Provence. Lavender is primarily used for perfume, aromatherapy, and tea—it is one of the most adored aromatic herbs in the world. It's cultivated in France, England, Europe, Africa, and the United States. It loves the sun and woody terrain. The official lavender is a shrubby herb with short, irregular stems, slender, straight leaves, and long-stemmed spires that bloom with whorls of tiny purple, aromatic flowers.

French lavender is the official medicinal herb, *Lavandula officinalis*. Spike lavender (called *lavender spica*) is found in mountainous areas of France and Spain, and this species is believed to be the lavender mentioned in the Bible as spikenard, with a fragrance that has a hint of rosemary. English lavender is a beautiful lavender known as *Lavandula vera*.

Lavender has a long history of use as healing water or rub in combination with other herbs. The Romans used it for therapeutic baths, and the first Queen Elizabeth in England took lavender tea as a headache remedy. It was one of the herbs in the queen of Hungary's healing water that was applied to her legs as a cure for paralysis, and it worked. In medieval England, lavender was used in bonfires to banish viruses, bacteria, and the plague. In France it was used to fight cholera. It is one of the herbs that the Pilgrims brought to the New World.

HEALTH VIRTUES: Lavender is antibacterial, antiseptic, calming, soothing, and a pain reliever and digestive aid. It's a tonic for the nerves and brain to reduce anxiety, tension, headaches, nervousness, mood swings, dizziness and fainting, vomiting, and diarrhea. It has a long tradition as an aromatherapy herb to lift the spirits and fight depression. Applied topically, it helps to ease pain and fatigue, cramps, and convulsions. It's a deodorizer, and a detoxifier for the spleen and liver, and it helps to lower blood pressure. Lavender has been used for skin conditions, including eczema, psoriasis, cuts, burns, swelling, and bruises. It's a potent antiseptic to fight infectious diseases and fevers; use it to clean the air in a sickroom. It was used in bonfires in the Middle Ages to fight diphtheria, typhoid, streptococcus, and pneumonia.

CULINARY PLEASURES: Only a dash of lavender is used in the herbes de Provence blend of France. Its best use is as tea and for aromatherapy. Place a vase of fresh lavender flowers on your table, or try lavender oil dotted on a windowsill when a breeze is coming in.

LEMON
Divine Rind

Citrus limonum, medica

PART USED: Rind, Fruit, Juice, Oil

Our lips will pucker as we taste a shred of lemon's yellow rind, and we'll go in search of a town in northern Italy that has been called paradise—Limone sul Garda, or Limone on Lake Garda—the largest lake in Italy. Here, the majestic Dolomite mountains surround the lake in heights that reach 8,000 feet. On the lower slopes, there are fertile hills for orchards and vineyards. A legend tells us that Saint Francis of Assisi visited the town of Limone in the thirteenth century and planted the first lemon trees. Five centuries later, 15 million lemons were produced, supported by rows of white stone columns that were connected by pine beams to form a frame at the top, which could be open-air in summer or closed off to shield the lemon trees in winter. It was known as a *limonaiae*.

The lemons from Limone were and still are considered the best in the world, but as the twentieth century dawned, lemons from Limone could not compete with cheaper and more prolific varieties in the market, which came from hotter climates where the lemon trees didn't require special care. Lemon production began its decline in Limone, and today, only a few arbors still thrive. Writer D. H. Lawrence described the scattered remains of the limonaiae columns from the lemon arbors as being like ". . . ruins of temples."

Known as Persian apples, lemons are one of the world's oldest fruits, and the tree is adored all over the world. It grows to an average height of eleven feet, with three colors on its bark: gray on the main trunk, green on the young branches, and purple-tinted twigs. It has bright green oval leaves with tapered tips, deep center spines, and serrated edges. The flowers are small pink blossoms with white interiors. The flowers are known as solitary flowers—only one small blossom announces the coming of the fruit. The fruit is oval-shaped, nippled at one end, smooth, bright yellow, and indented over the oil glands.

There are approximately fifty varieties of lemon trees, but *Citrus limonum* is the official herb, also called *Citrus medica*, presumed to be a native of India and Europe. The first mention of lemon was in 4000 BC in Pakistan. It was a Viking herb, and the English Queen Elizabeth I loved it in mead, a natural wine made from lemons, honey, spices, herbs, and water, fermented for three months and bottled like wine. America has Columbus to thank for its first lemon trees; on his second journey to America in 1493, Columbus brought lemon seeds.

HEALTH VIRTUES: The greatest power is in the slim outer skin of the rind of the lemon. It's for heart health, it's a blood cleanser, and it's a full body tonic. It's antiseptic, antibacterial, antirheumatic, and antioxidant. It's high in vitamin C and in bioflavenoids to strengthen veins, blood vessels, and capillaries; prevent thickening of arterial walls, bruising, and varicose veins; and promote healthy skin. It's a well-known infection fighter and fever reducer. Lemon also provides vitamins A, B_1, B_2, B_3, and mucilage (moisture). Lemon has an alkaline effect in the body to balance pH levels and remove acid wastes. Lemon tea is a time-honored treatment for coughs and colds. It's a purifier.

CULINARY PLEASURES: In Middle Eastern cuisine, lemon adds the zesty taste. A Lebanese favorite is lemon on boiled potatoes, and in Greece, boiled potatoes with lemon also include olive oil and oregano. In Germany, it's the tang in meatballs. In the United States, it's lemonade. Lemon brings spark to any fruit drink or tea and piques the flavor of sauces and meat, particularly lamb and fish.

CHOOSING YOUR LEMONS: Buy the heaviest lemons with the cleanest rinds. When you get the lemons home, grate off the thin, yellow outer skins and store them in a separate container. The volatile oil of lemon, the richest flavor, and the most potent health benefits are in this part of the rind. Store in the refrigerator with sprigs of parsley to keep them fresh longer. You can also freeze lemons and grate the rinds as you need them.

MARJORAM

Heart's Desire

Origanum marjorana (sweet)
Origanum vulgare (wild)
PART USED: Leaves, Oil

We will travel to the fifteenth century in Italy, to stand over the shoulder of a Dominican monk named Francesco Colonna, who is writing a story called *Hypnorotomachia*, which translates as Love's Struggle in a Dream. He is using a pseudonym, Polyphilius, and a series of gardens as a metaphor for the dream. One of the gardens begins with an outer circle bordered by clipped myrtle and cypress hedges. There are circles inside the outer circle, with different woodsy plants and trees in each circle: oaks, pines, rosemary, junipers, cypress, and laurel woods with bay.

The woods lead to meadows, with walkways and trellises for climbing jasmine, honeysuckle, and clematis. The corners of the meadows are planted with apple trees that are cultivated to form circles, growing on tiers with steps. On each step, a different herb is planted. Farther along, we see a garden with stone columns that is planted with aromatic herbs and shrubs, some in containers. In this garden, marjoram appears, and the whole area is enclosed by a rose garden that includes all of the roses that were described by the Roman naturalist Pliny. Farther along, we can see water and another meadow with flowering plants in every variety and color, including mint and marjoram. This garden in the Dominican monk's story is called "the garden of the heart's desire."

Marjoram is a member of the mint family that grows straight up, one to three feet tall on a hairy brown stem with a purple tint. The stems branch at the upper half, with small oval leaves in clusters. It flowers from June to October from the tips of its branches with exquisite purple flowers that have a hint of red. In Greece, if wild marjoram appeared on a gravesite, it was taken as a sign that the deceased was happy in paradise. In Greek and Roman weddings, the bride and groom wore marjoram wreaths to celebrate their happiness. Native to the Mediterranean, marjoram grows wild in Canada, and you can find it by roadsides all across the United States. You might spot it by chance, because marjoram's exquisite purple flowers may catch your eye, making you wonder, *What is that beautiful plant?* You can tell your companions in the car that it's one of the plants in the garden of the heart's desire. Marjoram is cultivated in Egypt, eastern Europe, France, and the United States.

HEALTH VIRTUES: Marjoram is an herb with a long history of use for stomach disorders and as a digestive aid. It's an antidote for poisons, a stimulant, and a tonic to ease nervous disorders including anxiety, headaches, and insomnia. It's also a remedy for phlegm, one of the four temperaments in the Greek model for healing, which was based on four elements that comprised the world: earth, air, water, and fire. These four elements corresponded with the four seasons, four bodily humors (fluids), and four temperaments. In each individual, one of the four temperaments could dominate, which could lead to health problems that the dominant temperament represented. A phlegmatic person had a cold and damp nature (waterlogged), which led to phlegm and chest problems. The goal was to restore balance of the four temperaments. Warm, drying herbs like marjoram were used to counteract the damp nature of phlegm and therefore restore balance.

CULINARY PLEASURES: The fragrance of marjoram lifts your spirits. It's an herb for blends, with a hint of mint and a lighthearted nature that blends beautifully with bay. It's one of the herbs used for accent in France's bouquet garni, and fines herbes. Use marjoram to inspire lightness in the heavier vegetables like cabbage and beans. It has a history of use in spice mixes for sausage—it is called the sausage herb in Germany. It's a popular seasoning for liver, and it also charms lamb, beef, pork, chicken, chowders, pickles, and salad dressings.

MINT

The Peppermint Cure

Mentha piperita (Peppermint)
Mentha spicata (Spearmint)
PART USED: Whole Plant, Flowers

In pursuit of peppermint, which is so popular in Britain, we'll check the London Pharmacopoeia in 1721, which listed peppermint as a medicinal herb. Then we'll visit the peppermint district: Mitcham in Surrey, where, as early as 1750, aromatic peppermint broke the ground with its purple-tinted stem, smooth green, spear-shaped leaves with serrated edges, and tiny red-violet flowers that bloomed from spikes in dense whorls. At the time only a few acres in Mitcham were allotted to medicinal plants, but peppermint was so adored in England that fifty years later, peppermint had staked its claim (with underground runners) on more than a hundred acres in Mitcham. This presented a problem because there were no stills at Mitcham in the 1800s to extract the peppermint oil, which meant that the herb would have to travel by train to London for processing. A train trip for a fresh-picked herb required special considerations for harvesting and travel so the herb wouldn't lost its potency, and peppermint was so valued that Maud Grieve, in *A Modern Herbal*, recommended late afternoon harvesting and a night train to London for peppermint. That way, the herb could travel in the cool of the evening.

The peppermint crop in Mitcham expanded to 500 acres by 1850, and other areas in England began to cultivate mint. To this day, Mitcham is known as the premier peppermint district for growing and distilling mint and had its followers; a peppermint district in Italy became known as "the Mitcham of Italy."

Peppermint has been beloved around the world from ancient to modern times, used as a medicine, food, strewing herb for fragrance, to fight bacteria in the air, in wreaths for noble heads, and even to repel mice—since mice won't come near an area that contains peppermint. Japanese men often carried peppermint in small silver boxes that hung from their belts. It would give them energy and purify the air around them.

HEALTH VIRTUES: Peppermint is a tonic herb that is considered a cure-all. It's antiseptic, analgesic, astringent, a decongestant, a pain reliever, a digestive aid with a calming nature, and a *nervine* to strengthen the nervous system, ease stress, depression, and calm you all over. The menthol in oil of peppermint has an anesthetic effect on nerve endings in the stomach, which stops nausea and seasickness. One whiff of the fragrance is a pick-me-up. Taken as a tea, peppermint can ward off colds and infections; it fights congestion in the chest and can clear nasal passages. It has been used for palpitations of the heart, colic, dyspepsia, flatulence, and in baths to combat body odor. It has a healthy supply of nutrient and antioxidants that include vitamins A, B-complex, and C (flavenoids), carotenoids, betaine, choline, minerals, tocopherols, phytol, azulene, and the vital oil of peppermint, which is the third most poplar oil in the world after lemon and orange.

Peppermint is cultivated in France (known as red mint), with a higher yield of oil, but the oil is not as potent as English peppermint. Sicilian and Italian peppermint are rated on a similar scale with English peppermint. It is also cultivated in North America.

Spearmint. Most experts agree that this is the mint that grew in the Holy Land and was mentioned in the Bible. Universally treasured, it grows wild all over the world with square stems, short stalks, spear-shaped leaves that are bright green and wrinkled, with finely toothed edges and very prominent middle seams (ribs). It flowers in whorls of pink or lilac. Spearmint was loved by the ancient Greeks, who combined it with lemon balm and other herbs for baths to calm and strengthen the nerves and sinews. The Romans brought it to Britain, where Chaucer wrote of its charming nature. The health virtues of spearmint are similar to peppermint, but milder.

CULINARY PLEASURES: Spearmint is generally considered the best mint for cooking, but it's all a matter of taste. Mint is the lift in Greek meatballs and classic Middle Eastern dishes. It's a standard herb for lamb, peas, jellies, jams, new potatoes, salads, and teas. See chapter 22 for peppermint and spearmint in high-energy iced teas.

MUSTARD
The Stimulant

Brassica family
PART USED: Seeds

To appreciate the importance of this spice in France during the reign of Louis XI, we'll look in on the royal court to find everyone in a tizzy. The king will be traveling. Where is the royal mustard pot? King Louis XI wouldn't leave home without it.

Mustard got its name from the method that was used to produce it. The seeds were ground into a paste and blended with must, an unfermented wine. It is one of the oldest spices in the world, made from members of the *Brassica* family who are as varied as families can be in physical appearance, but they have one common denominator: hot seeds.

White mustard seeds were used 2,000 years ago in the Han dynasty in China. Mustard was a favorite of ancient Greeks, who attributed its creation to Asclepius, the god of healing. It was recommended by Hippocrates as a poultice for muscle pains since it stimulates circulation to the area and helps to draw out toxins, and it is still considered one of the best poultices today, especially for sciatica. The ancient Romans used it for pickling and flavoring.

White Mustard (*Brassica alba, Brassica hirta*). White mustard comes in hairy pods with hard, round, light-beige seeds, and the outer skin removed. Hotness scale is medium.

Black Mustard (*Brassica nigra*). Black mustard has long seedpods with seeds that can range from brown to deep brown. It's stronger than white mustard, and it's considered the most pungent mustard.

Brown Mustard (*Brassica juncea*). The seeds are similar in appearance to black mustard, but it falls midway between white and black mustard for pungency. Also called Indian mustard.

MUSTARD BLENDS

All-American Ballpark Mustard. Contains the ancient white mustard seeds, sugar, vinegar, and turmeric, the sacred root from India, for coloring. It's mildly hot mustard.

Standard American Yellow Mustard. Contains white mustard seeds, vinegar, salt, turmeric, and often paprika and garlic powder. It's mild but zesty.

Bordeaux Mustard. Contains unhusked black mustard seeds and unfermented wine, often flavored with tarragon. Dark brown mustard. Strong.

Dijon Mustard. A blend of husked black mustard seeds, spices, salt, and wine, and it can range from mild to hot, and vary in tints of yellow-brown. It's a must in French mustard sauces and salad dressings.

English Mustard. Contains white mustard seeds, often mixed with wheat flour and turmeric for color. Hot.

German Mustard. This mustard can vary in strength, depending on the vinegar that is added to the blend. It contains black mustard seeds and vinegar in various strengths. Smooth.

Meaux Mustard. Contains half ground and half crushed black mustard seeds and vinegar. Hot and crunchy.

HEALTH VIRTUES: Mustard is a stimulant that increases blood flow, and a diuretic, which helps to remove toxins from the body. It increases the production of gastric juices to serve as a digestive aid, and it's a natural laxative. It's a good spice for constipation and respiratory conditions. Black mustard is an aphrodisiac and blood purifier. It's worth noting that the turmeric in mustard blends is the golden root that helps to fight cancer.

CULINARY PLEASURES: Mustard is an ingredient in Indian ghee. The powdered form is used commercially as an emulsifier in salad dressings, mayonnaise, barbecue sauces, and baked beans. It's a popular spread for sandwiches and a standard for spice blends that are used to marinate meat and seafood.

NUTMEG (and MACE)
The Enhancer

Myristica fragrans

PART USED: Dried Seed Kernels

We will raise our eggnog glasses and tip them for a toast to the camel, often described as the most cantankerous animal ever to succumb to the whims of man. And yet the ancient spice trade depended on the camel to cross the Arabian deserts from the Persian Gulf to the Mediterranean Sea, carrying spices from distant lands. It is believed that this ancient form of trade dates back to the origins of civilization.

Imagine that we are sitting on a dune in the Arabian desert, with nothing but sand on all sides as far as our eyes can see. Suddenly we think we are hearing bells like chimes from a temple. Out of nowhere, camels appear, traveling in a line, bound together—tail to head—carrying sacks tied with hand-woven bands in brightly colored stripes. The lead camel is decorated with beads and bells. Guides lead the camels on foot, while others ride on horseback, wearing robes that are dyed with colors from the spices. The procession of camels passes before our eyes like a mystical dream.

It is an Arabian caravan of the spice traders in ancient times. A string of fifty camels might be seen traveling alone in ancient times, but more often, a group of strings would travel together for safety. All told, several thousand camels could be crossing the desert at one time, stretching for miles. The camels carried exotic peppers, cloves, cardamom, indigo, musk from China, nutmeg and mace from India, Persian coffee, and the roots of many other spices and herbs.

There were no roads or specified routes, only the instincts of the guides, who used the traditional routes that were traveled by their fathers before them, to cross the vast desert sands. To prepare for a caravan, merchants would gather their own camels and others that were hired for the journey. The caravan would be guided by a leader who was paid for his services. They timed their walks to avoid the heat of midday, starting before dawn, stopping before noon, moving again in the early afternoon until late in the evening, when they stopped for the night and cooked the main meal of their day. Walking at a camel's pace—two miles per hour—the caravan could cover twenty-eight miles on a good day, and the journey could take months. Homing pigeons would be sent ahead to gauge the progress of the caravan, with relay stations for the pigeons at fifty-mile intervals.

The lands of Arabia produced no spices, and yet the world's greatest spices from unknown lands crossed the Arabian deserts with the Arab traders. The exact routes of the ancient spice trade have never been fully confirmed, lending an air of mystique to the caravans of Arabia to this day.

The home of the nutmeg and mace carried by the camels was the Mollucas, known as the Spice Islands, on the southwestern coast of India. The nutmeg tree can reach twenty-five feet in height, with a smooth, gray-green bark that is oily (yellow). It branches in whorls, with dark green, glossy elliptical leaves that can be four to six inches long. It flowers with male and female blossoms. The male flowers are pale yellow, with three erect teeth. The female flowers are similar but solitary. The tree only blooms after nine years of age and continues to fruit for seventy-five years.

The nutmeg fruit is a succulent drupe, blotchy yellow, and edible. When the fruit is split, there is a bright red netty covering over the seed—called the aril—which is dried and sold as mace. The nutmeg seed is found under the aril, encased in a dark, shiny, oval shell. The seed is approximately one inch and oval, fleshy and brown on the outside, with a paler brown inside. The fruit is gathered three times a year, the mace is separated from the nut, and the nutmeg and mace are dried separately. Nutmegs are often sun-dried for a week, then dried for three to six weeks over a slow charcoal fire. When the seeds are dried, they rattle in their shells like castanets. The shell is cracked, and the nutmegs are graded for potency. Small, round, heavy nutmeg seeds are considered the best. Larger, longer, lighter, and less oily seeds are considered inferior. The properties of mace and nutmeg are the same.

Nutmeg was attributed magical powers and worn as amulets to ward off disease. In Europe, men often carried silver, ivory, or wooden graters that contained nutmegs, since nutmeg was known as a spice for virility and to attract admirers. Connecticut is often called the Nutmeg State, reminiscent of the days when salesmen sold wooden carvings of nutmegs as charms against evil.

HEALTH VIRTUES: Nutmeg is an aromatic spice that lifts the spirits and heightens the senses. It is also a spice for a calm stomach, digestive ease, and intestinal health, since it increases digestive enzymes and helps to prevent fermentation of undigested food in the intestines. It's cleansing for the liver, spleen, and joints.

CULINARY PLEASURES: Nutmeg lends an exotic flavor to eggnog and mulled wines. It is often combined with cinnamon for sweet custards, puddings, pies, cookies, and spice cakes. A popular companion for cheese in soufflés and sauces, nutmeg is an ingredient in Italian mortadella sausages, Middle Eastern lamb dishes, and Moroccan spice blends.

USING NUTMEG SEEDS: The flavor of nutmeg seeds fades quickly, making whole nuts the preferred way to keep nutmeg fresh, using a grater for each use. The whole nuts have an indefinite shelf life, but the nuts and ground nutmeg should be stored in airtight containers in a cool, dark place. **A note of caution:** Large doses of nutmeg can cause hallucinations. Keep nutmeg out of the reach of children and avoid serving dishes or drinks with nutmeg to children. The recommended use of nutmeg is culinary amounts: usually a pinch from a fresh seed, or one quarter to one half teaspoon dried nutmeg in a whole pie or spiced dish. In large amounts, nutmeg can be fatal. One nutmeg equals two to three teaspoons of ground nutmeg, and, for some people, two to three whole nuts or six to nine teaspoons taken at one time can be a lethal dose. If you take medications, check with your doctor before using nutmeg, since it is not known how nutmeg interacts with medications.

USING MACE: Mace has similar properties to nutmeg and dries to a lighter color than nutmeg, making it the preferred form of nutmeg in lighter-colored dishes like custard and cream sauces.

OREGANO
The Tonic

Origanum vulgare

PART USED: Leaves, Stems

We're following a group of American soldiers stationed in Italy in World War II. They're going to lunch, and they order pizza. Later that afternoon, we see the same soldiers having a snack. You guessed it, pizza! The pie that originated in Lebanon was dressed up in Italy, but what was it that made Italian pizza so tantalizing? You guessed it, oregano! In World War II, when American soldiers were stationed in Italy, pizza mania was born. Prior to World War II, there was no record of oregano imports on U.S. customs lists. When soldiers returned home, they complained like crazy: "Why don't we have oregano?" It made its debut in the United States to achieve instant fame. Oregano bloomed in gardens, graced open-air markets, and was dried for herbal shakers. The result was a 5,000 percent increase in U.S. sales of oregano since the war. That's a lot of oregano.

Oregano is a woody perennial that can reach three feet in height. It has a square stem with a reddish tint and seamed elliptical leaves, and it blooms in clusters of dark pink blossoms. It's a native of Europe and loves to live by the sea.

HEALTH VIRTUES: Oregano is a stimulant, with a warm, drying nature. It's also a tonic for energy and an expectorant for chest congestion. It has a long history of use as a digestive aid to ease stomach discomfort. It has a mild tranquilizing effect on the nervous system, to ease nervous tension. It removes toxins from the body, and fights colds, flu, and fevers. Its volatile oil contains carvacrol and thymol, which are antibacterial and antifungal. Oregano has been used as a scalp wash to stimulate hair growth. It is often confused with wild marjoram, but oregano's properties are stronger than marjoram's and should be used more sparingly.

CULINARY PLEASURES: Oregano is popular in Italian, Greek, South American, and Spanish cuisine. It's the herb for pizza and tomatoes, often combined with basil, and it's one of the herbs that can be found in chile powder. Oregano adds zest to cheese dishes, sauces, stuffing for fish and meat, peas, potatoes, corn, and vegetable and beef broth. The fresh leaves are vivid in salads. A must for Italian green beans.

PARSLEY
Green Goddess

Carum or Apium petroselinum
PART USED: **Leaves, Root, Seed**

Let's visit a food market to select the variety of parsley that will provide the best flavor and texture for our everyday cooking needs. Two basic varieties are cultivated for food: root parsley and leaf parsley. Root parsleys include Hamburg parsley—often called turnip-rooted parsley, which has a root that you can eat as a vegetable. Leaf parsleys include Neopolitan—often called celery-leaf parsley, and the leaves and stalks can be eaten as a vegetable. There are many varieties of curly leafed parsley, but plain flat-leafed parsley is generally considered the best parsley for cooking. Be on the lookout—in most markets cilantro is displayed next to parsley and cilantro leaves are strikingly similar to flat-leafed parsley, so it's easy to pick up cilantro by mistake if you don't check the tags on flat-leafed parsley.

Parsley's origins are presumed to be eastern Mediterranean. It's an herb that loves to grow on walls and rocks, with thick white roots, dark green leaves, and white flowers. Its average height is a foot tall.

It was cultivated in England as early as 1548 and naturalized in

Scotland, where it grows on ancient walls and rocks. It was used in Greece to crown victors and feed chariot horses.

HEALTH VIRTUES: Parsley is an antioxidant and tonic herb that helps to fight cancer. It also has a cleansing nature for healthy glands, including the pituitary, thyroid, adrenal, lymph, prostate, and swollen glands. It's a mild antibiotic for immune system strength. Parsley is also a natural antihistamine; it suppresses histamine production, and that makes parsley valuable for allergies, asthma, hives, and headaches, which have been linked to high histamine levels in the blood. It's an oxygenator for the cells with chlorophyll; it's high in potassium (antitumor) and a tonic for the heart, promoting healthy arteries and capillaries to reduce high blood pressure. Cleansing and diuretic for a healthy bladder, parsley is also a blood builder and natural anti-inflammatory—for any disease that ends in *itis*, which means *inflamed*. It's an herb for healthy vision, and it fights gout, rheumatism, sciatica, and varicose veins. It's a digestive stimulant and the best breath freshener—it counters garlic. Parsley is one-fourth protein and contains vitamins A, B-complex, B_1, B_2, and B_3. It is high in vitamin C, iron, and calcium (fights polyps) and also contains sodium, sulfur (health protector), silicon (healthy skin, hair, nails, vibrancy), cobalt, and selenium.

CULINARY PLEASURES: Parsley is a favorite all over the world and is the most popular herb in the United States. It is used freely in salads and finely chopped for soup, stuffing, sauces, dips, and blends from the simple to the exotic.

PAPRIKA Known as Hungarian pepper and Spanish pepper. See Pepper.

PEPPER
Master Spice

Piper nigrum

PART USED: Fruit (Peppercorns)

We are looking for the origin of a spice that was once worth more than gold. To find its essence, we will have to listen to the whispers of the monsoon winds and follow them back in time to the forests of southwestern India on the Malabar Coast—4,000 years ago. Here we are told about a seed capsule with five compartments and five spikes at the top of each compartment. It grows on a vine from the buttercup family, with grayish green leaves and white flowers with blue veins that have five petals on each flower. If we find one of these capsules, it will be like finding a pearl.

The Arab spice traders found the capsules of peppercorn in India and brought them to the Phoenician merchants who dominated the trade routes that would take pepper from the East to the lands in the West. The legends of the spice trade were rooted in the East, where most of the great spices of the world originated—and the story of the spice trade is often called the story of pepper, the master spice. The Arab traders told tales of wild elephants that roamed in the mist of the East and fragrances that wafted in the winds like perfume from paradise. The desire for pepper and other spices of the East took on a mythical status as the quest for paradise. Eden was thought to be a real garden in the world that could be found in the East, behind the curtain of mist from the monsoon rains. The aromatic fragrances and tastes of the spices from India only enhanced that belief.

This dream of paradise in the East was promoted by the spice traders for a very practical reason: to maintain control of the spice market, in order to keep the prices high. The higher the price of pepper rose in Western lands, the greater the demand for pepper grew. To own pepper was to own a gift from paradise. The Arab traders saw the potential for wealth beyond measure in the booming pepper trade, if they could do two important things: keep the origins of the spices and the trade routes secret and remove the middlemen, the Phoenicians. Over time, that's exactly what the Arab traders did. They alleged that the origins of the spices were Arabia, not India, and they told stories about the treacherous monsoon winds that could make a camel's hair stand on end, making the journey to the East seem dangerous and forbidding.

The Arabian tales of the origin of the spices appealed to the Greeks in the fifth century BC, who were dream spinners themselves, but the Greeks were as practical as the Arabs when it came to acquiring riches. While they promoted the Arabic tales about the origin of the spices, the Greeks set about finding their own route to India to cut out the Arab middlemen.

The Roman historian Pliny was more practical about the matter of spices. He estimated that the Arab monopoly of pepper increased its price 100 times from the price of origin, and the lands of the East were bleeding Rome. The Romans set about finding their own route to India to cut out the Arab middlemen, which was vital to the Roman economy, since Romans were known as the most insatiable consumers of aromatic spices in the world. Rome even tried an invasion of Arabia in 24 BC to break the pepper monopoly, but it was a dismal failure.

In the dawn of the first century under the Roman calendar AD, a miracle happened. A Greek merchant uncovered the secret of the monsoon winds that the Arab traders had been withholding. The winds reversed direction in the middle of the year, which meant that trips from Egypt (on the Red Sea) to southwestern India in midyear would not be long and dangerous; they would be relatively easy. With this revelation, the Arab monopoly on spices was broken, and the Romans dealt directly with the Egyptians in Alexandria to trade with India, cutting out the Arab middlemen. Rome reaped the profits from the spice trade for 600 years, expanding her empire in the West, where pepper was welcomed with a passion.

But Rome's independence in the spice trade didn't last. The Arabs had been regrouping to regain control of the trade routes, and 641 AD proved to be a turning point. The Arabs conquered Alexandria, Rome's door to the East. A tariff was imposed on pepper for Europe that equaled a third of the price of all of the spices that passed through Alexandria. Pepper became a spice that was only affordable in Europe by the rich. Dowries included pepper; debts were paid in pepper; it was used like gold.

The merchants of Venice stepped into the fray and made a deal with the Arabs in Alexandria that gave Venice all but exclusive control over the spices that reached Europe. Wealth from the pepper trade shifted to Venice, which became one of the richest and most luxurious cities in the world, with marble palaces and Oriental influences in its design to show visitors that the merchants of Venice had powerful friends.

The only hope for the pepper-crazed Europeans was to find a sea route to India, to search for the Spice Islands by water, using a gateway called Malacca, which turned out to be a fable. Spain and Portugal suffered great losses looking for the fabled gate, but then Vasco da Gama rounded the Cape of Good Hope to reach India by way of Africa in 1498, and the Portuguese traders returned home to Lisbon with cargoes of spices, including the master spice, pepper. To the dismay of the Venetians and their partners in Alexandria, the price of pepper in Portugal fell to one-fifth the price in Venice, and the Europeans were penetrating the mist of the East again.

The Spaniards, meanwhile, were not entirely pleased that Christopher Columbus had discovered a New World instead of the route to the Spice Islands. He had returned to Spain with chile pods that he called red pepper, believing that any cargo of pepper would be heralded as a success. But it was not the pungent, aromatic black pepper from the Spice Islands, and it wasn't really a pepper, but the name pepper stuck to the chile pods, creating confusion about the names of the peppers that remains to this day.

A complicated struggle for dominance in the pepper trade contin-ued in Europe, with Portugal maintaining a slim hold, while other merchants, like the Dutch East India Company, were creating havoc in the East, fighting for control of pepper.

Meanwhile, the Pilgrims had left England to colonize the New World, and Salem, Massachusetts, became the first American port to toss its Yankee chips into the pepper trade. It seemed impossible for the Yankees to triumph over the distances that had to be traveled for America to compete in the pepper trade, but it's exactly what they did. The first clipper ship was designed, and when it set sail for for-eign ports, it proved to be the fastest ship in the world. The first mil-lionaire in America was created from the pepper trade.

HEALTH VIRTUES: Pepper is a hot, aromatic spice with antibacterial virtues to fight infections. It's also a stimulant that increases circula-tion, which cleanses the body of toxins, reduces the oxidation of fats, strengthens the liver and spleen, and helps to prevent premature ag-ing and susceptibility to disease. It stimulates the taste buds and the production of digestive enzymes to improve digestion and ease bloat-ing and gas. It is known to ease nausea. It warms the stomach and in-creases the body temperature to fight chills and fevers. Because of its cleansing nature, it has been used to fight respiratory ailments, tu-mors, and cystic conditions. It's a spice to use for cold hands and feet.

CULINARY PLEASURES: Pepper stimulates the taste buds, which en-hances the flavor of any food it is used on.

Freshly ground pepper is an experience in flavor, aroma, and taste. It is at its best ground directly onto the food at the table with a pep-per mill. When pepper is used to flavor heated foods, it's best to add it just as the food comes off the heat to maintain pepper's aroma. Whole peppercorns have a long shelf life when they are stored in an airtight container in a cool, dark place. Once the pepper seeds are broken, the aroma and heat will fade quickly.

Preground pepper has only the barest hint of an aroma and very minimal heat. It cannot match the taste of freshly ground pepper, but most people like it anyway. *Coarsely ground pepper* is available in a shaker, and it falls midway between whole pepper and preground pepper for flavor and texture.

KNOW YOUR PEPPERS

Black Pepper. The berries are picked before they ripen and are dried. They blacken as they dry. It's the most popular pepper.

White Pepper. The berries are left on the vines longer to ripen the berry cores. When they are picked, the berries are soaked in water to soften the outer shell so it can be removed. The result is a whiter pepper with a milder heat rating, commonly used in white sauces.

Green Pepper. The berries are picked before they mature, often used in green sauces for fish, on green vegetables, and in soups with greens.

PEPPERS FROM OTHER PLANTS

Paprika (Capsicum annum). A mild red pepper with a sweet nature that is used for different varieties of paprika. It is known as Hungarian pepper and Spanish pepper, and it is cultivated in Hungary, Spain, South America, and California. Paprika gives Hungarian cooking its unique flavor—think of chicken paprikash and Hungarian goulash. Columbus brought paprika to Spain from America on his second voyage, and there is a smoked paprika in Spain called *pimenton*— think of Spanish sausage (chorizo and lomo pork loin), and think of paella. In the United States, paprika makes you think of deviled eggs and kebabs.

Chipotle Chile Pepper (Capsicum annum). Made from Mexican chile peppers (jalapeños), this pepper is smoky and sweet with moderate to high heat.

Ancho Chile Pepper (Capsicum annum). Made from Mexican chile peppers (poblanos), it has a mild, sweet, paprika flavor with moderate heat, and it's one of the chile peppers used in the well-known Mexican mole blends.

POPPY SEEDS
Seeds of Tranquillity

Papaver somniferum

PART USED: Seeds

This herbal adventure takes us back to 1609 in the Netherlands, when the Dutch gained their freedom from Spanish occupation, and the Dutch renaissance began. A renaissance in gardens began as well. The walls around Dutch gardens could become freer, since they were no longer needed as protection from the Spanish invaders.

We find canals of water (moats) for natural barriers, instead of walls. Beyond the canals, we see orchards and vegetable gardens that are separated from the farmlands by other canals. The gardens themselves retain a classical outline: a rectangle subdivided into smaller rectangles and squares, which are plots for planting, but they are less restricted by their relationship to the main house or castle; they are freer to be art forms in themselves. We can take a shady stroll under trees planted between the plots, with arbors or fountains at cross points of the paths, and we can delight in the fragrances and colors in bed after bed of decorative flowers.

If we could see this garden from above, we would realize that we are walking in an intricate maze, like the gardens that were illustrated in the prints of Hans Vredeman de Vries, a sixteenth-century architect. The beds of brightly colored flowers might include sunflowers, like the ones painted by Vincent van Gogh, African marigolds, roses as a symbol of Christianity, and the ancient and mysterious flowers with the exotic looking capsule—the poppy, known today as the Holland poppy.

The annual poppy is a tall, stately herb that can reach six feet, with strong, round stems and large green leaves that have a silvery glint. The large poppy flowers can range in color from a reddish purple to pink and pure white. The capsules are round with a depression at the top, and contain rays of the stigma with a ring below, where the capsule meets the stem. The capsule also has an exotic appearance and can vary in size, but some have been known to grow as large as an apple.

Before the seed capsule matures, cuts are made in the walls of the poppy capsule, and a milky alkaloid substance is removed and dried. This is the source of the opiate properties of poppy. The seeds and oil don't develop until after the milky alkaloid is removed, and it is generally agreed that poppy seeds have no narcotic properties. The kidney-shaped seeds are minute and plentiful in one capsule, and they range in color from slate blue to white.

The poppy flower is a symbol of honor, with a long tradition as a tribute to fallen warriors. In World War II, when Canadian soldiers freed the Netherlands from Nazi rule, one of the soldiers sat on the rear step of an ambulance and wrote a poem about poppies that grew among the crosses that marked the gravesites of Canadian soldiers. He never expected it to become a world-famous poem, used in history classes—in "In Flanders Fields." Wild poppies have been known to grow in fields where heroes died.

The native lands of the poppy are presumed to be India, China, Turkey, and Iran. It was one of the earliest plants in history to be cultivated in Europe, and today it is cultivated around the world, but Holland and Canada are considered the main producers of poppy seeds.

HEALTH VIRTUES: The seeds have a calming nature. They have been used as a sleep aid, to ease restlessness and stomach discomfort, and to treat respiratory problems, bronchitis, asthma, hoarseness, coughs, sinus conditions, and gout.

CULINARY PLEASURES: Poppy seeds have a mellow, nutty flavor and aroma. In India, the seeds are coated with sugar to make candy, and ground poppy seeds are used as thickener for sauces. The seeds are an ingredient in fragrant Jewish cakes and breads, and in vegetable, noodle, and fish dishes. They're popular in German dishes, cultivated in Egypt as a source of cooking oil, and used as an ingredient in the Japanese spice blend, *shichimi togarashi*, along with Szechuan pepper for a subtle, nutty taste. Turkish desserts often contain ground poppy seeds.

USING POPPY SEEDS: Poppy seeds need heat to release their nutty flavor and provide a crunchy texture. The heat in baking or simmering will accomplish this, but if you are using the seeds in salads, salad dressings, or as a garnish, burst the flavor by baking the seeds in a 350-degree oven for fifteen minutes, or you can quickly panfry poppy seeds in butter.

ROSEMARY
The Revitalizer

Rosmarinus officinalis
PART USED: Whole plant

Where shall we go to find this piney perfume? Let's go sailing along the Mediterranean coast in the morning dew and moor in France to look for a small shrub with woody stems and dark green narrow leaves that resemble pine needles. This evergreen member of the mint family will make us feel invigorated each time we break off a leaf and inhale its fragrance.

Rosemary was used in ancient Egypt for wall gardens, to perfume and cleanse the air. In Rome, it was used as a hedge around formal gardens and as crowns in festivals. It was a treasured herb in monastery gardens in England. In Hungary, a bottle of healing water contained rosemary, lavender, and myrtle, and was sold by vendors as Queen of Hungary's Water—from the blend that was used by the queen of Hungary to cure her paralysis—and she attributed the cure to rosemary. Brides, including royal brides, often carried rosemary in bouquets or entwined it in the crown of their veils as a symbol of love. Greek students often wore rosemary wreaths on their heads during exams to improve their memories. It was one of the herbs that were used to avert the evil eye, which meant illness in the Middle Ages. One legend claims that the Virgin Mary tossed her cloak over a rosemary bush when she stopped to rest, and the next morning, the white flowers had turned to blue.

Rosemary has a long history of use as an incense and disinfectant. It was burned in hospital wards in France to help to prevent the spread of infectious diseases. As a strewing herb, it was used to perfume the air and ward off insects.

HEALTH VIRTUES: Simply inhale the fragrance or taste a fresh leaf on your tongue, and you'll feel invigorated in an instant. This is an herb to move chi, the vital energy of life. It's a circulatory tonic for energy and vitality, to strengthen the memory and brain, and to maintain a healthy heart and blood pressure. It fights the circulatory problems that accompany diabetes by improving circulation to the legs to alleviate puffiness. This herb has many virtues to fight infections and inflammatory diseases. It's a natural anti-inflammatory, antiseptic for cleansing, antiviral, and antimicrobial, with antioxidants and flavonoids to prevent premature aging. It's also a decongestant and mild expectorant for respiratory health. It's a digestive aid and a *nervine*, an herb that eases stress and fights depression. It's a vital herb to help to restore immunity and health. Rosemary tea applied to the scalp stimulates circulation to revitalize the hair. Some say it can even re-store hair loss. Rosemary also helps to burn fats.

CULINARY PLEASURES: Rosemary was used to season meat in ancient Greece. It's a rich seasoning for chicken, lamb, fish, soups, stews, and salads. It harmonizes well with zucchini, green beans, and as-paragus, and it is bliss on Brie. See chapter 11, "Sandwich Haven," for a Brie and rosemary grilled sandwich. Fresh rosemary leaves will give you the best flavor and taste. If you use dried rosemary in cold dishes, grind the leaves with a mortar and pestle first, because the dried leaves can be brittle. Rosemary is potent, so use it sparingly.

SAFFRON
Threads of Mystique

Crocus sativus

PART USED: Flower Stigmas

Our search for the saffron crocus with slender green leaves, purple petals, and an intoxicating fragrance will be like a magic carpet ride to flowering fields in the ancient world.

We begin with ancient Persia (current-day Iran), where the land is dry and the mountains high, absorbing most of the water from the rains. And yet, in early summer, an array of crocuses appear for a short time in the parched valley, to sing of beauty. Persia is presumed to be the native land of saffron (*za'farān*), the most expensive spice in the world. However, because of the harsh growing conditions and the volume of flowers that are needed to produce one ounce of saf-fron, Persian saffron never achieved prominence in the marketplaces of the world.

We travel southwest to ancient Assyria (current-day Iraq), where saffron was used as a medicine, and on to Phoenicia (current-day Syria and Lebanon), where the traders took saffron wherever they went. We move onward to India, where saffron was used as a medi-cine, food, and as a dye for Buddhist robes.

We sojourn in ancient Crete, where it is believed that this member of the lily family grew in prehistoric times, since excavations in Knossos unearthed a fresco called the "saffron gatherer," showing a monkey carefully walking between yellow crocus blossoms. In Greece, where many herbs were romanticized to mythical status, saffron had its own unrequited-love story.

Legend tells us that the crocus was named for a young mortal named Crocus, who fell in love with a nymph, Smilax, only to be rebuffed by her. Upon her death, young Crocus suffered such despair and longing for her that he was transformed into a crocus for eternity. The crocus flower was associated with fertility in ancient Greece; Hippocrates and other Greek physicians used saffron as a therapeutic medicine. The poet Homer captured the essence of the saffron crocus, which blooms at night, filling the air with its aphrodisiac perfume. Homer described morning as "the crocus veil" of dawn.

The ancient Romans are credited with bringing saffron to England, where another myth was born. Saffron was adored in England, but after the Dark Ages, the crocus wasn't seen on the English landscape anymore. A story is told about a pilgrim to the Holy Land who concealed one crocus bulb in a hollow staff and brought it back to England, under penalty of death. (Odd how this story reminds us of Prometheus hiding fire in the hollow staff of fennel.) That one crocus is believed to be the mother of all of the crocuses in England today. It was cultivated with abandon in a town called Saffron Essex, whose coat of arms depicts three saffron crocuses.

It might be mentioned here that the saffron crocus is unique, and it's not a good idea for us to pick a crocus from the wilds to have a taste of saffron before we continue our journey. Some varieties of crocuses are toxic, and we could fall off our magic carpet before we reach our final destination, Spain, the major producer of saffron in the world today. We are going to a town that is known for a legend of eternal love and enchantment in literature, La Mancha.

The home of *The Man of La Mancha* is also the home of saffron in Spain. It seems quite magical, doesn't it? We are told that it takes 75,000 blossoms to make one pound of saffron, since there are only three stigmas in each flower, and the stigmas must be gathered by hand, daily, when the flower opens. We are sure that the saffron gatherers don't mind the work. The scent of thousands of blooming crocuses would be aromatic bliss. It could make you believe that the Garden of Eden is in the here and now.

Saffron is cultivated in Greece (known as red saffron), Turkey, India, France, Italy, and the People's Republic of China.

HEALTH VIRTUES: Saffron is one of the spices that are considered cure-alls. It has an exhilarating nature and rejuvenating properties. It increases circulation, which makes saffron a full-body tonic for heart health, vitality, and defense against toxins accumulating in muscles and joints. It contains vitamins A and B_2, calcium, potassium, phosphorus, and sodium.

CULINARY PLEASURES: Adored all over the world and particularly in England, saffron is especially nice in rice and spectacular in Spanish paella. See chapter 19, "Make a Little Magic with Fish," for A Very Special Paella recipe that gives you step-by-step directions.

USING SAFFRON THREADS: Saffron yields its properties to boiling water; therefore, it's best to soak a few threads (stigmas) in water and add the liquid to your dish at the end of cooking. You can't use dry threads in cold or dry dishes, but you can toss them into a soup or stew that has liquid, since the water will release the properties. You can also dry roast the threads before infusing them in water to enhance the flavor. Use with a delicate hand. Only one or two threads of saffron are needed for an entire rice dish. If you use dried saffron, be sure to purchase it from a reputable source, since dried saffron can be adulterated with other herbs to provide a yellow color.

SAGE
Eternal Sprit

Salvia officinalis

PART USED: Leaves, Root

In our search for the wisdom of the sages, we will bridle a palomino and follow our Indian guide to the western plains in the early days of America. We will ride through the many varieties of wild sages, with their blooming spires, some with silvery leaves and flowers in hues of every purple we can desire, some with crinkled greens and burnished red or chocolate blossoms, and others with pebbled leaves and spires of ultramarine or cobalt. The fragrance of sage will waft around us and work its charm, to make us feel calmer and more centered, less up in the mind and more in the moment. That is the nature of sage, known as the herb of wisdom and longevity.

Sage is known as a sacred herb and was regarded as a cure-all. It was so adored by the masters of herbal wisdom, the Chinese, that they traded tea for European sage and imported American sage.

Among the many beautiful sages, *Salvia officinalis* is a perennial that can reach two feet in height, with square stems and wooly leaves that are grayish green and oblong. From June to September, whorls of violet-blue flowers bloom from the top of the stem and branches.

Sage grew in Jerusalem (*Salvia judaica*), where its growth pattern inspired the design of the seven-branched candlestick of the Hebrew religion. It has a long history of use as incense to cleanse the air or consecrate sacred places. In the Italian medical school at Salerno, this quotation was featured: "Why should a man die who grows sage in his garden?"

HEALTH VIRTUES: Sage has health virtues that support the claim that it is the herb of wisdom and longevity. Antibiotic, antioxidant, antifungal, antiseptic, astringent, cooling (it will break fevers), and calming, it is a circulatory stimulant that also offers vital energy from vitamins A, B_1, B_2, B_3, C, and E, calcium, iron, magnesium, manganese, phosphorus, potassium, selenium, silicon, sodium, sulfur, and zinc. In China, sage is used to enhance vital energy and as a heart herb. It helps to revitalize every system in your body from head to toe. It's an excellent herb for stress, confusion, insomnia, and all nervous disorders. It cuts the fat in food. It's totally wholesome.

CULINARY PLEASURES: Sage is popular in the United States and one of the most versatile herbs. Use it with meats (especially turkey), soups, sauces, casseroles, stuffing, salads, jellies, potatoes, bread, beans, rice, and any bland vegetable. It's the main ingredient in Bell's Seasoning, the Thanksgiving blend. Use sparingly; a little goes a long way.

SAVORY (Summer)
Warming Ease

Satureja hortensis

PART USED: Leaves

We will visit "the gardens left behind," in the notes of John Josselyn, one of the early American settlers. He compiled a list of plants that the colonists brought to America to remind them of the English gardens they had to leave. Among the herbs was summer savory, an aromatic member of the mint family of savory, which includes fourteen species. Summer savory is an annual with slender, woody stems and hairy, oblong green leaves that have a tint of brown. It blooms with pale lilac flowers.

Legends say that savory belonged to the Satyrs, the half-man, half-goat forest deities who attended Bacchus, the god of wine and wantonness. Perhaps they needed savory to help him recover from his excesses. The poet Virgil grew savory as nectar for his bees, to get a richer honey. In England, Shakespeare mentioned savory in *The Winter's Tale*.

Savory is native to the Mediterranean, cultivated in France, the Balkans, and Yugoslavia, which is considered to produce the premier grade.

HEALTH VIRTUES: Aromatic summer savory is a calming digestive aid with a warming nature. In England, it's a classic remedy for colic and a cure for flatulence. It's also an expectorant for phlegm. It may contain thymol and carvacrol, which would give savory antioxidant properties. It was used in history as a poultice with wheat flour for sciatica and palsy. A leaf rubbed on the skin was used for relief from a wasp or bee sting.

CULINARY USES: Summer savory is commonly used in blends with thyme and marjoram. It's hotter and drier than winter savory. It was used like pepper in the early days of the United States, before pepper could be imported. In ancient Rome, it was used to flavor vinegar. In the Middle Ages in Europe, savory was an ingredient in cakes, pies, puddings, stuffing, sausages, pork pies, and pea soup. Known as the bean herb, savory is a standard in Germany for all bean dishes. Savory is often used as a substitute for parsley.

Winter Savory is similar to summer savory, but it has a stronger taste. Known in England since 1562, it was mixed with bread crumbs to flavor meats and fish, specifically trout. It's less popular than summer savory for culinary use and isn't mentioned medicinally. Native to the Mediterranean, winter savory was introduced to England by the Romans and migrated to the United States with the Pilgrims.

STAR ANISE
Anise of the East

Illicium verum
PART USED: **Seeds**

This journey will take us to the East, to see if the rocks and water in a Mandarin garden will tell us a story. The essence of Chinese gardens is shan shui, which means "mountains and water." The rocks suggest the solid nature of mountains or yang, the masculine principle. The flowing water suggests yin, the feminine principle. The rocks are often placed so their reflection can be seen in the water, since yin and yang each contain a seed of the other. The movement of the water is also an essential aspect of the garden, and the movement tells its own story.

We see water cascading down a hill into a pool below that separates into several streams. Each stream will take its own course. One has found its way to a solitary arch in the distance that is encircled with sand and brightly colored pebbles, and the stream flows around the arch to create the illusion of an island. Two streams have found their way to a meadow, where one forms canals while the other forms pools, and they weave in and out, around each other, in a fluid dance. Often, the streams meet rocks that impede their progress, and the friction creates waves that form new streams to seek new directions. In these gardens, there are many suggestions of obstacles and new directions. Amid a dense planting of bamboo, we find a path that leads us to a flowering herbal garden in a valley, and if by chance we should look up while we walk, we will see pavilions where we least expect them, calling us to climb and stand under their protection to see the next horizon.

We are looking for an evergreen tree from the magnolia family that can grow to thirty feet, with leaves like blades, pale yellow flowers, and a most unusual, rough-skinned, rust-colored fruit—an eight-pointed star. The stars are seedpods that can be more than an inch long. They are picked and dried before the fruit can ripen to preserve the intense licorice flavor—like anise but more pungent. Star anise doesn't come from the same plant family as anise, but it is known as the anise of the East.

HEALTH VIRTUES: Star anise is a calming spice to relieve digestive stress and relax the muscles of the digestive system to ease spasms, indigestion, and gas. It is used in Chinese medicine for rheumatism, back pain, and hernias. It is considered safe for children to relieve colic.

CULINARY PLEASURES: Star anise provides a touch of the East for duck and poultry, simmered chicken and beef dishes, chicken stocks, and soups. In China, it is often chewed whole as a breath freshener and digestive aid. In the West, it is often used instead of anise for liquors that are digestive aids. If you use star anise instead of anise, begin with lighter measures, since it is more potent.

HOW TO USE THE STARS: Star anise is available in whole stars, segments, or as a ground powder that is a coppery brown color. The stars can be stored whole in airtight containers for at least a year without losing their flavor. Whole stars can be used in simmering dishes or ground to a powder prior to use, segment by segment.

TARRAGON
Little Dragon

Artemisia dracunculus
PARTS USED: Leaves, Stems

Let's take a medieval escape to the days of knights and dragons and doe-eyed maidens on an August afternoon, when tarragon will be blooming. We are looking for a member of the sunflower family, a fragrant bush about two to three feet tall, with woody stems and spear-shaped grayish green leaves that are delicate to the touch. Its small, round flowers will be yellow and black, but we'll have to look closely at the flowers, since they rarely open.

Aromatic tarragon is a legendary herb known as little dragon or herb of the dragon in many languages. In the Middle Ages, special powers were attributed to the dragon herbs—they could repel dragons and snakes, and were regarded as antidotes for venomous stings and the bites of mad dogs. In a modern translation, the myth could mean that the dragon herbs helped to remove toxins from the body. Tarragon also carries the blessing of the moon goddess Artemis in its name. With this lineage, it's no surprise that tarragon was used as incense to consecrate holy places, and it was carried as a charm or in sachet pouches for good luck.

Tales of tarragon date back to Greece in 500 BC. Hippocrates used it as a simple, which means a one-herb remedy. As it migrated west, tarragon was grown in French monastery gardens and English royal gardens in the time of the Tudors; it continued to migrate west to America in the early 1800s. An old folk tale recommends putting tarragon in your shoes for a long journey to insure stamina, which makes sense if you put the tarragon under your socks, next to bare feet, since herbal properties can be absorbed through the skin.

HEALTH VIRTUES: True to its dragon lore, tarragon has a cleansing, diuretic nature that helps to eliminate toxins from the body, particularly the undigested by-products of red meats and meat proteins that can cause intestinal discomfort, bloating, gas, and water retention. In addition to being a calming digestive aid, tarragon is an herb for a healthy heart, with rutin, a bioflavenoid that helps to keep plaque from clinging to artery walls. Its volatile oil eugenol is anaesthetic to fight pain. It's refreshing to the taste and very energizing.

CULINARY PLEASURES: There are three types of tarragon in culinary use: French, Russian, and Mexican. Of the tarragons, French tarragon (also called German tarragon) is considered the best tarragon with the richest flavor. It's one of the herbs in bouquet garni. Tarragon is at its best when it is used fresh, since the volatile oil is lost in drying. However, you can freeze fresh tarragon to preserve its virtues; just ignore the darker color of the leaves. Toss the leaves into salads for a rich fragrance and flavor. Use tarragon vinegar in cream sauces and mustard sauces; it's the ingredient that gives béarnaise, hollandaise, white mustard, and French mustard blends their special character. Try it on rice—it's nice. The whole herb can be cut just above the stems and frozen to preserve its freshness.

THYME
Mother Thyme

Thymus vulgaris
PART USED: Leaves, Flowers, Stems

On this journey, we are traveling back in time in search of a fragrance that Kipling called "dawn in Paradise." We've heard whispers that the herb can be found in a bed in a manger where a woman named Mary gave birth to a son called Jesus. We will follow three men who are traveling there with gifts of gold, myrrh, and the herbal incense frankincense, to a manger in Jerusalem, where Christianity was born.

Legends say if you sleep on a bed of thyme and inhale its fragrance, it will cure depression and epilepsy, you'll never have nightmares, and you'll wake feeling exhilarated. Thyme represented courage and bravery in ancient Greece and was used for strength, vitality, and clarity of mind, and was burned as incense to clear the air of illness and disease. In the Middle Ages, when knights were going into battle, the women would embroider scarves with a design of a honeybee and a sprig of thyme to give to the knights for protection and to bring them home safely.

HEALTH VIRTUES: Thyme is truly dawn in paradise when it comes to fighting infections. It's a natural antibiotic, antiviral, antifungal, antibacterial, and antiseptic. It is especially good for the respiratory tract, where the breath of life is maintained. It's a bronchodilator and cleanser, an expectorant to reduce phlegm (a source of infections), and a chest decongestant. It's a shield to fight invaders from colds, flu, viruses, and respiratory diseases. The Greeks were on target to use thyme for clarity of mind, since it clears your head, throat, chest, and lungs to improve airflow through your body. Its antiseptic fragrance can clear the air in a sickroom and fight fevers. It's also a vital herb to cleanse the kidneys and urinary tract and to fight infections that can linger. It calms and soothes the digestive system. It's been used for treatment of uterine disorders.

CULINARY PLEASURES: Thyme is one of the herbs in bouquet garni, often used in combination with parsley and bay. It brings a sweet balsamic flavor to meat, fish, and poultry dishes. I never cook red meat or chicken without it. Toss it into sauces, stews, stuffing, meat, poultry, soups, and salads. Take it as a tea for recovery from illness or at the onset of any infection.

TURMERIC
Culinary Gold

Curcuma longa

PART USED: Rhizome

We are dreaming of India, where an aromatic spice from the ginger family has been revered for 4,000 years as culinary gold. We are looking for the rough-skinned root of a plant with long-stemmed, bright green leaves and clusters of pale yellow ornamental flowers. Known as *holdi* in India, the root we call turmeric is derived from Latin *terra merita*, which means "meritorious earth," for the tint of gold in its root. A golden color in the root of an herb will often grant the herb a special privilege, since gold is linked with divinity and royalty, and that is true for turmeric, a holy herb in India. It holds a place of honor to this day as the spice that dyes the golden robes in Hindu religious ceremonies.

The powdered yellow spice we use in our kitchens comes from turmeric's rhizomes, which are fingerlike stems from its root that are boiled, dried, and polished for sale in the marketplace. It is known as yellow root in many countries where it is cultivated, but its country of origin is presumed to be India. It dates back 4,000 years to the Vedic culture, and Ayurvedic (life-knowledge) medicine, which equates illness with imbalance and uses herbs and dietary changes to restore balance. As a holy herb, turmeric is added to every dish in India, including meat, potatoes, beans, and vegetables. Since 600 BC, it has been used as a medicine, flavoring, and dye, and it is still used today in wedding rituals as a body dye.

When Marco Polo found turmeric in his travels, he refered to it as a "vegetable" with the properties of saffron, and it is often called Indian saffron, but it shouldn't be taken as a replacement for saffron, which is a completely different herb. India produces the world's largest supply of turmeric and uses the majority of it. It is also cultivated in China, Taiwan, Java, the Philippines, Haiti, Jamaica, and Peru.

HEALTH VIRTUES: It's a touch of gold in your menu, with powerful antioxidant and anti-inflammatory properties (curcumin) to fight cancer and degenerative diseases. Laboratory studies show that curcumin can inhibit the growth of cancer cells in vitro, and it appears to block the buildup of beta-amyloid, which is believed to be a major factor in the cause of Alzheimer's disease. It's a calming digestive aid with a ginger fragrance and a pungent flavor that has a hint of orange. It stimulates bile to digest fats, and protects the liver from damaging toxins. It's also an anti-inflammatory herb (termerone), to fight diseases of inflammation (any disease that ends in -*itis*, such as arthritis, cystitis, hepatitis). Its antibacterial nature makes it an infection fighter, especially in the glands, and it has been used to fight leukemia, lymphoma, and HIV viruses. It's a heart herb, too, with anticholesterol properties to lower cholesterol, help to prevent strokes, and combat blood clots. It has been used to treat intestinal parasites and to regulate menses.

In Chinese medicine, turmeric is linked with the liver, heart, and lung channels, and is used to promote the flow of chi—vital energy— to move the blood, calm the nerves, quiet the mind, and clear heat from the heart to relieve depression. It stops hemorrhaging, dissolves clots, and is used to treat hepatitis and encephalitis.

CULINARY PLEASURES: When you want a hint of eastern mystique in western cuisine, turmeric is the herb to choose. It's the spice that gives Indonesian rice its yellow tint and exotic flavor, and it's a mandatory ingredient in curry. Use sparingly at first, since the light, ginger aroma is a mask for a taste that can seem bitter or musky. To lighten the musk effect, use a splash of lemon. It is excellent with chicken, rice and beans, in stews and sauces, and to charm vegetarian cuisine. It's part of the yellow curry paste of Thailand, where it is made from a fresh rhizome. It's used in Vietnamese sauces and popular in Ethiopian cuisine, where it is called long pepper. Turmeric is also popular in sauces, relishes, mustards, pickles, and chutneys.

VANILLA
Sweet Nectar

Vanilla planifolia
PART USED: Beans

We are searching for a bean from an orchid that is called the "nectar of the gods" as we follow a band of Spanish adventurers, led by Hernan Cortes, through a mountain pass that leads to a deep valley in central Mexico. It is November 1519. They reach the clearing, gaze into the valley below, and see something they can hardly believe.

A great white city is floating on a glistening lake, connected to the shores by three linear causeways with canals, footpaths, and wide roads that converge on a central area where temples and pyramids tower over the city. The city is immaculate, gleaming with white-wash, colored stucco, and rooftop-gardens, and is four times larger than Seville. The Spaniards call the city an "enchanted vision." Some of Cortés's men will later write that they weren't sure it wasn't a dream.

It is the city of Tenochtitlan, ruled by Montezuma II, built by the Aztec/Mexica people—a composite of several tribes of nomads who had lived on the fringes of society until they put down roots on islands in Lake Texcoco, in the central basin of Mexico (current site of Mexico City). They claimed that a divine vision from their gods chose this site for their city.

The Spaniards are welcomed into the city as ambassadors and given a tour of the city. They are stunned to see that everything in the interior of the city is immaculate as well: there is no visible dirt or grit, and the people are immaculate. They are told that this is a sacred city where sweeping honors the gods. There are public latrines, with a chain of canoes along the canals to remove the waste for fertilizer. They see floating gardens in the canals, which provide corn, fruit, and flowers for the people. The palaces of the lords are as elegant as the palaces of the Moors, with courtyards, pools, and draperies in the halls. All of the people are soft-spoken, mannerly, and pious—even the warriors, who are dressed in full regalia. The priests seem similar to the Spanish priests who have traveled with Cortés—lean and pious, dressed in long, black robes.

During their months in the city, the Spaniards keep detailed records about every aspect of this sophisticated culture. It includes a system for agriculture that is ecologically based, laws that are strictly enforced, a working system of taxation, written language and copious records, and a highly stratified social order that is so complex, it is difficult for the Spaniards to comprehend. But the Spaniards also see the dark side of the empire: sacrifices to the gods that are performed by the priests and warriors on a daily basis, and on some occasions, thousands in one day. The illusion of the white city becomes like a nightmare to the Catholic soldiers. They leave the city after eight months with a vow to return and take this empire down stone by stone, no matter how long it takes.

The Spaniards did return several times for a period of two years and gained the support of local allies, who shared their fear of the Aztec/Mexica empire and its power in the region. They brought down the empire and returned to Spain with beans from two plants they found in the region. It was a discovery made by Bernal Diaz, one of Cortés's men, who had asked Montezuma what the ingredients were in the chocolate drink he enjoyed. One ingredient was cocoa, and the other was vanilla. The nectar of the gods was on its way to Europe for the first time.

Europeans went wild for the exotic fragrance and taste of vanilla, but to their dismay, they couldn't cultivate the vines in tropical climates outside of Mexico. The orchids had to be pollinated by hummingbirds and bees that were found only in Mexico. Mexico remained the leading producer of vanilla for the next three centuries, until 1841, when a technique for artificial pollination was discovered, and vanilla began to thrive in islands of the West Indies.

The herb is a tropical orchid that wraps itself around trees or poles to support itself. The flowers begin as narrow bells encircled by thin petals, and for several months, they elongate into narrow seedpods. The pods are picked green and can be dried in the sun, heated in an oven, or cured in hot water, which causes the glucosides to break down into glucose, forming a crystalline component that was named vanillin—the pure vanilla that charmed the world.

HEALTH VIRTUES: Vanilla has health-protecting properties that support its earliest claim as a nectar. It's an antioxidant, which makes it a free radical scavenger that defends the body against premature aging and diseases, including heart disease and cancer. It's also a stimulant, which improves circulation and increases vitality. It's an aromatic spice, which lifts the spirit, and it's a *nervine*, which soothes the central nervous system and fights nerve-related disorders, including depression. It also fights fevers and has been used to treat hysteria and impotence.

CULINARY PLEASURES: Vanilla is the spice for sweetening, used in pudding, pies, cakes, muffins, chocolate filling for eclairs, fudge for hot fudge sundaes, sweet drinks . . . a world of sweets.

Whole Vanilla Beans are the best way to experience the pure taste of vanilla. To use, split the bean's pod and scrape out the seeds with a sharp knife for each use. Bake the seeds in an oven, keeping watch until they release their fragrance, or soak them in hot water until the oil is released. Don't refrigerate the beans. Wrap them in plastic and store them in an airtight glass jar or plastic bag. Many people retain the pods to use to sweeten lighter fare.

Pure Vanilla Extract is produced by cutting the beans into small pieces and soaking them several times in hot alcohol. The bottle will proudly display its ingredients, since the process of extraction is time-consuming and respected. The ingredients will be water, alcohol, and extracts of vanilla beans.

Imitation Vanilla Extract is known as adulterated vanilla, which imitates the flavor of vanilla with a variety of ingredients, but it doesn't contain real vanillin from real vanilla beans. It is usually packaged in a box that looks like the extract box, so be observant.

Three primary vanilla beans are popular in the market today:

Madagascar Bourbon (Vanilla planifolia). Long, slender beans, with thick, oily skins, lots of tiny seeds, and a rich vanilla flavor and aroma.

Mexican (Vanilla planifolia). Similar in appearance to Madagascar Bourbon beans, but smoother, more mellow, and with a spicier fragrance.

Tahitian: The most expensive beans, considered the best. Shorter, plumper beans with thinner skins, fewer seeds, and a higher content of oil and water than Madagascar or Mexican beans, with a fruitier fragrance.

WATERCRESS
The Invigorator

Nasturtium officinale
PART USED: Leaves, Roots

We've traveled to many gardens, and it seems fitting that our last adventure takes us on a walk by a quiet stream to find a member of the mustard family with a mildly pungent taste. Watercress is a delicate plant with dark or pale green leaves that can be found growing wild by brooks and streams. It symbolizes stability.

HEALTH VIRTUES: Watercress is a tonic herb and a blood purifier with fabulous nutrition. High in vitamins A, C, and E—the antioxidants—which are also anti-inflammatory, it also has iron for blood building, calcium for the bones and prevention of intestinal polyps, phosphorus, iodine for a healthy thyroid, copper, sulfur, and nitrogen. It strengthens the heart, liver, kidneys, and thyroid, and it's a blessing for the skin, to fight all skin infections, including acne, eczema, and ringworm. The juice can be used directly on the skin for eruptions. Watercress is an excellent herb to fight the depleting effects of stress and to overcome mental and physical exhaustion. It's a great vitality herb for seniors.

CULINARY PLEASURES: Use freely in salads, sandwiches, soups, stews, and vegetable medleys. Chew it for instant pep.

CHAPTER 3

Buying and Storing Your Herbs and Spices

Fresh herbs are the best cooking pleasure, especially those that are organically grown as close to home as possible, from local or regional organic farms that take pride in their growing standards and advertise them. Open-air markets are fabulous resources, but talk to the vendor to find out where the herbs were grown and what standards were used, and get the information you need to feel confident that the growing conditions for the herbs meet your satisfaction. Pick up the herbs you are planning to buy, and carefully look them over before buying.

Many fresh herbs are available year-round in supermarkets and natural food grocery stores, but basil in winter is never quite like basil in the summer. Remember to buy lots of basil at the end of the summer and freeze the fresh leaves in olive oil in ice cube trays covered with clear wrap or in plastic airtight containers. You can also dry fresh basil just enough to take the moisture out and stack the leaves in a plastic container in the freezer, to use one or two at a time all winter long. The leaves will retain their flavor, but you have to ignore the splotchy dark black color.

Wash fresh herbs thoroughly before refrigerating them, remove the brown or defective-looking leaves, and store them in foil or wrap with a spray of mist to keep them plump. Use fresh herbs as soon as possible after buying them. Make sauces and dips to have on hand for fresh herbal snacks. Fresh parsley will last longer if you store it in a jar of water in a compartment on the door of your refrigerator, where it will greet you with its vivid green energy when you open the door.

Fresh dried herbs are the next best for cooking, and again, local or regionally grown herbs are an excellent choice for fresh dried herbs, since there is a shorter transportation time from the source to your kitchen. Fresh dried herbs should be stored in airtight, dark-colored containers in a cool, dark place, since heat and light will reduce their potency. Buy fresh dried herbs in small amounts so you will use them up quickly and replace them frequently.

I buy fresh dried herbs from a Vermont grower who ships by mail, but only after I visited the location and saw the quality for myself. With a little investigation, you can find a local or regional supplier who will meet every expectation.

Shaker herbs and spices have convenience as their advantage, and most people rely on this version for seasoning. When you are buying dried herbs and spices in shakers, you want only the natural herb or spice, not salt, sugar, or unnecessary additives. This lets you control the sugar and salt in your menu, rather than finding them in an herb by surprise. You can add a lot of unnecessary sugar, salt, and additives to your system without realizing it, unless you check the ingredients of every shaker herb you buy.

Many herbs come in salt versions, such as garlic salt, celery salt, or parsley salt. You want the true herb only—garlic, celery seed, or parsley—not the salt versions, which will mask the flavor of the true herb and add unnecessary salt to your menu. If there are no ingredients listed on the shaker, buy another brand, because you can't be certain about the contents.

Shaker blends call for a little extra attention to the ingredients label. Blends can vary with the herbs and spices they use, but many blends can include sugar, salt, and MSG, which can cause headaches (sometimes severe), a feverish feeling, and heart throbbing, and in excessive amounts can be harmful to the heart and brain. MSG has no flavor, so check the ingredients carefully. A blend of chile powder, for instance, should be a blend of peppers, natural dried herbs and spices, and may include binders such as carotene, but shouldn't include sugar, salt, or MSG—and I found several blends that had them. The best lemon pepper shouldn't contain sugar or added salt. Be especially observant with Thai blends; they often contain sugar and MSG, which are preferred ingredients in Thailand, but you can find versions of Thai blends without them. If the shaker blend doesn't include a list of the ingredients, use another brand, since blends are easy to adulterate by using other herbs that imitate the color.

The most reputable shaker herbs are the ones that indicate the ingredients clearly on the label, and there are many fine brands to give you a wide selection. Experiment with different brands until you find the one that really pleases you.

I wouldn't recommend buying blends that are sold loose, unless you know the supplier and can trust that person wholeheartedly. Saffron is often sold loose, but I wouldn't recommend buying it that way, since you don't know what you're getting. Make the investment in bottled saffron with a manufacturer that stands behind the label. Good saffron is worth the price, and a little goes a long way.

Whole dried seeds of spices have different requirements for different seeds, which you can find in "Nature's Bouquet of Healing Herbs and Spices for Cooking" under the name of each spice.

If you buy herbs and spices on the Web, place small orders at first, so you can gauge the quality of the product before making a bigger investment.

Most of all, enjoy the experience of investigating herbs and spices. The knowledge you will gain is worth the time and effort, and it can result in many delightful discoveries. The one thing I've learned about herbs and spices is that you can never learn enough about them. The more you learn about them, the more you love and admire their charm and individuality and the pleasure they add to your menu. Then one day, you realize how much they've enhanced your life, and you'll know what all of the great herbalists know about the herbs and spices and their vital health benefits: They love you back.

Freezing Herbs

Before you freeze fresh herbs, wash them and blanch them in a small amount of boiling water for a few minutes, and immediately set them in ice water to cool them. Drain the ice water, place the herbs in a freezer container, and freeze them. You can remove a few leaves at a time and thaw them for use. Basil and parsley freeze best as purees. Puree parsley or basil in a chopper with just enough water to make a smooth blend, and freeze the puree in a covered ice cube tray. Pop a few cubes from the tray to use like fresh parsley or basil.

CHAPTER 4

The All-Naturals Guide

The following chart is your guide to the healing benefits of the herbs and spices for cooking. At a glance, you can find natural antacids, natural antibiotics, natural antioxidants, and the top-notch herbs and spices to use in your everyday menu for natural health support. It's also a vital resource you can use to target specific herbs and spices for specific health issues you'd like to improve.

ANTACID

Caraway	Celery Seed	Fennel

ANTIAGING

Allspice	Basil	Cayenne	Celery Seed
Chives	Cloves	Dill	Fennel
Garlic	Ginger	Horseradish	Lemon
Parsley	Peppermint	Rosemary	Sage
Spearmint	Tarragon	Turmeric	Vanilla
Watercress			

ANTIBACTERIAL

Bay	Basil	Caraway	Cayenne
Chives	Cloves	Coriander	Garlic
Oregano	Pepper	Thyme	Turmeric

ANTIBIOTIC

Garlic	Parsley	Sage	Thyme

ANTIFUNGAL

Bay	Cayenne	Cinnamon	Coriander
Garlic	Oregano	Sage	Thyme

ANTIHISTAMINE

Parsley

ANTI-INFLAMMATORY

Anise	Cayenne	Cloves	Dill
Fennel	Garlic	Ginger	Lemon
Parsley	Rosemary	Sage	Turmeric
Watercress			

ANTIOXIDANT

Anise	Allspice	Basil	Cayenne
Celery Seed	Chives	Cloves	Dill
Fennel	Garlic	Ginger	Horseradish
Lemon	Parsley	Peppermint	Rosemary
Sage	Spearmint	Tarragon	Turmeric
Vanilla	Watercress		

ANTISEPTIC (CLEANSER)

Basil	Cayenne	Celery Seed	Cinnamon
Cloves	Fennel	Garlic	Ginger
Horseradish	Lemon	Peppermint	Rosemary
Sage	Spearmint		

ANTIVIRAL

Cayenne	Cinnamon	Garlic	Ginger
Rosemary	Thyme		

ARTHRITIS AID

Allspice	Bay	Cayenne	Celery Seed
Chives	Coriander	Ginger	Horseradish
Lemon	Parsley	Star Anise	Turmeric

ASTHMA AID

Anise	Garlic	Oregano	Savory
Thyme			

BLOOD BUILDER

Basil	Cayenne	Celery Seed	Chives
Fennel	Parsley	Sage	Watercress

BLOOD CLEANSING

Lemon	Mustard	Watercress

BLOOD PRESSURE REDUCTION

Bay	Celery Seed	Chervil	Chives
Cinnamon	Garlic		

BLOOD SUGAR REDUCTION

Cayenne	Celery Seed	Cinnamon	Coriander
Dill	Garlic		

CALMING
See Tension and Stress Relief.

CANCER FIGHTER
(ANTIOXIDANTS AND ANTIOXIDANT COMPOUNDS)

Allspice	Basil	Cayenne	Celery Seed
Chives	Cloves	Dill	Fennel
Garlic	Ginger	Horseradish	Lemon
Parsley	Peppermint	Rosemary	Sage
Spearmint	Tarragon	Turmeric	Vanilla

CHOLESTEROL REDUCTION

Chives	Coriander	Garlic	Ginger
Turmeric			

CIRCULATION

Basil	Cayenne	Cinnamon	Fennel
Ginger	Mustard	Oregano	Parsley
Pepper	Rosemary	Saffron	Sage
Vanilla			

COLDS, FLU, AND RESPIRATORY INFECTIONS
See Antiseptic, Antiviral, Decongestant, Expectorant, and Respiratory Strength.

CONSTIPATION
See Digestive Strength.

DECONGESTANT

Marjoram	Peppermint	Spearmint	Thyme

DEPRESSION FIGHTER

Basil	Chervil	Cloves	Coriander
Dill	Parsley	Rosemary	Saffron
Thyme	Turmeric	Vanilla	

Also see Digestive Strength, since digestion disorders can be a source of discomfort that feeds depression. Also see Nervous System Support.

DIABETES FIGHTER
See Blood Sugar Reduction and Circulation.

DIGESTIVE STRENGTH

Anise	Allspice	Caraway	Cardamom
Cayenne	Celery Seeds	Chervil	Chives
Cinnamon	Cloves	Coriander	Cumin
Dill	Fennel	Ginger	Horseradish
Marjoram	Nutmeg	Oregano	Parsley
Pepper	Peppermint	Savory	Spearmint
Star Anise	Tarragon	Turmeric	

EXPECTORANT

Anise	Chervil	Garlic	Horseradish
Oregano	Rosemary	Savory	Thyme

FAT FIGHTER

Cayenne	Chives	Fennel	Garlic
Ginger	Pepper	Rosemary	Turmeric

FEVER REDUCTION

Cayenne	Lemon	Oregano	Pepper
Sage	Vanilla		

GLANDS (HEALTHY)

Cayenne	Chives	Garlic	Ginger
Parsley	Turmeric	Watercress	

HEART HEALTH

Bay	Cayenne	Chives	Cinnamon
Dill	Garlic	Ginger	Lemon
Parsley	Peppermint	Rosemary	Sage
Spearmint	Tarragon	Turmeric	Vanilla
Watercress			

INDIGESTION
See Digestive Strength.

IMMUNE SYSTEM STRENGTH

Bay	Basil	Caraway	Cayenne
Chives	Cloves	Coriander	Garlic
Oregano	Parsley	Pepper	Rosemary
Thyme	Turmeric		

INSOMNIA AID

Dill	Poppy Seeds	Sage	Thyme

LAXATIVE

Horseradish	Mustard

NAUSEA, VERTIGO, MOTION SICKNESS

Ginger	Pepper	Peppermint	Spearmint

NERVOUS SYSTEM SUPPORT

Basil	Bay	Cardamom	Caraway
Celery Seed	Chives	Coriander	Dill
Oregano	Peppermint	Sage	Spearmint
Vanilla	Watercress		

PARASITES (ANTIMICROBIAL)

Garlic	Cloves

PAIN RELIEF

Anise	Caraway	Cayenne	Cloves
Dill	Peppermint	Spearmint	Star Anise
Tarragon			

PUFFINESS AND BLOATING

Dill	Fennel	Horseradish	Rosemary

Also see Circulation and Digestive Strength, since better circulation and digestive system strength can ease common water retention problems.

RESPIRATORY STRENGTH

Anise	Bay	Chervil	Cinnamon
Dill	Garlic	Ginger	Horseradish
Lemon	Mustard	Oregano	Pepper
Poppy Seeds	Rosemary	Thyme	

RHEUMATISM AID

Bay	Cayenne	Chives	Coriander
Ginger	Horseradish	Lemon	Parsley
Star Anise	Turmeric		

Also see Antiseptic to cleanse toxins and wastes to ease rheumatic aches.

SKIN HEALTH

Chives	Lemon	Watercress

Also see Antiseptic and any herb or spice with sulfur.

SPIRIT LIFTING

Cardamom	Chervil	Cloves	Coriander
Dill	Marjoram	Nutmeg	Peppermint
Rosemary	Saffron	Spearmint	Vanilla

TENSION AND STRESS RELIEF

Basil	Bay	Caraway	Cardamom
Celery Seed	Chives	Coriander	Dill
Oregano	Peppermint	Sage	Spearmint
Vanilla	Watercress		

TOXIN AND WASTE CLEANSING (FIGHTS INFECTIONS)

Basil	Cayenne	Celery Seed	Cinnamon
Cloves	Fennel	Garlic	Ginger
Horseradish	Lemon	Peppermint	Rosemary
Sage	Spearmint		

THYROID SUPPORT

Garlic	Watercress

VISION (HEALTHY)

Caraway   Fennel   Parsley

PART II

The Magic Teaspoon Recipes

CHAPTER 5

A Fresh Start

Four vital essentials can make a big difference in your health: parsley, lemon, garlic, and olive oil. To reap the health benefits of herbs and spices in your menu, you don't have to revamp your entire life or change everything you cook and eat in one sweep. If you begin by using fresh parsley, fresh lemons, fresh garlic, and extra virgin olive oil, you will be amazed at the healing power you can gain from these four remarkable gifts from Mother Nature. Keep them on hand at all times—and try to use parsley, lemon, and garlic fresh, even if you use the other herbs and spices dried.

Fresh Parsley: the Green Goddess of Health

Parsley is a potent antioxidant and tonic herb with a cleansing nature for healthy glands—pituitary, thyroid, adrenal, lymph, and prostate. It contains a mild antibiotic for immune system strength, and it's an antihistamine to fight allergies, asthma, hives, and headaches, conditions that have been linked to high histamine levels in the blood. It's an excellent source of chlorophyll, which oxygenates the blood, and it contains vital compounds that help to fight cancer. With fresh parsley, you are receiving herbal support for a healthy heart, arteries, and capillaries, to fight high blood pressure. It's cleansing and diuretic for a healthy bladder, and it's a natural anti-inflammatory for diseases that end in *itis*, which means *inflamed*. Parsley is packed with nutrients that include the vitamin B-complex, B_1, B_2, B_3, sodium, sulfur (the health protector), silicon, cobalt, selenium, and potassium. It also gives you 2 grams of protein, 114 mg of calcium, and 4,760 IU of vitamin A (antioxidant) in one cup. It's the best breath freshener.

For your personal health bouquet, keep fresh parsley on hand as your first vital cooking essential. It's the best thing you can do for your health.

Fresh Lemons and Rinds: a Four-Star Healer

Lemon is the fruit of the tree *Citrus limon*, with powerful healing properties. Using fresh lemon is an important step you can take toward a healthier life and greater pleasure in your daily menu. Nothing can match the taste and flavor of fresh lemon for cooking, and lemon has a vivid, cleansing nature to remove toxins from the body. It reduces fevers and fights colds and flu. The lemon may seem acidic, but its nature is alkaline in the body, to fight acidic conditions and remove acid wastes—vital for arthritis. Lemon is antiseptic, antibacterial, antioxidant, and high in vitamin C and bioflavonoids to strengthen veins, blood vessels, and capillaries; prevent thickening of arterial walls, bruising, and varicose veins; and fight infections. It provides vitamins A, B_1, B_2, B_3, and mucilage (a moisturizer). Lemon and honey tea is a time-honored treatment for coughs, colds, and bronchial conditions.

Take the time to save the rinds. The rind of the lemon—the slender covering of yellow—contains one of the most popular oils in the world, the volatile oil of lemon, which has the richest flavor and the most potent health benefits in the lemon. Freeze your lemons after you have used the juice, and grate the rinds or peel them off when you need them, being careful not to include the white area just below the rind, which is bitter. Sprinkle grated rind on vegetables, meat, chicken, and fish, or in sauces and dips; use slivers in fruit drinks and iced teas, or pop one in your mouth instead of candy to get a refreshing, cleansing lift. Use them every day! That way, you'll be getting a steady supply of a heart and skin herb, blood cleanser, and full-body tonic. It can't get easier than this to give yourself a gift of greater health.

Choosing your lemons: the heaviest lemons with clean, unbroken rinds are the best.

Fresh Garlic: a Health Tonic

Keep fresh garlic cloves at your fingertips for everyday use. Fresh garlic has a rich flavor that mellows in cooking, and it provides powerful healing benefits.

Known as a heal-all, garlic was used in Egypt 4,000 years ago for strength and endurance, heart problems, respiratory problems, and to fight tumors. It was used by Hippocrates and taken as a stimulant by Greek athletes before competitions. In Russia it is known as Russian penicillin, because it contains a natural antibiotic with the strength of penicillin and no side effects. It's antiviral, antifungal, antibacterial, and antiseptic, and it kills parasites. Garlic is also an immune system stimulant to fight infections. It increases the production of interferon in the body, which is a defense against cancer, and it contains selenium and germanium, which are also anticancer. It's an antidiabetic herb that helps to reduce blood sugar and a heart tonic with an anticlotting agent; it helps to lower cholesterol, reduce hypertension, and fight high blood pressure. Garlic also contains enzymes that protect the liver from toxins, including lead. It's an antiaging herb and a free radical scavenger. Its health benefits have been extensively researched in Japan, Germany, and the United States. It's for healthy glands, including the lymph glands and thyroid.

Garlic is a good source of sulfur, which guards your health. It also contains phosphorus, potassium, manganese, zinc, calcium, magnesium, sodium, iron, copper, vitamins A, B-complex, and C, and amino acid proteins. It increases metabolic heat, which helps to burn fat. Use it for energy, to fight fatigue, to speed recovery from illness, and to foster healthy glands. It promotes wound healing. It's also an expectorant for phlegm.

I've heard some people say that they don't eat garlic because they don't want garlic breath. No problem! To counter garlic breath, chew parsley, and add parsley to dishes that contain garlic.

Extra Virgin Olive Oil: the Oil with Antioxidants

Extra virgin olive oil is the heart-smart oil to use in your daily menu. It has very low acidity and provides all of the health benefits of olives, which are high in antioxidants to protect cells from free radical damage and premature aging. No other oil is as rich in monounsaturated fatty acids, which help to control bad cholesterol (LDL) and increase good cholesterol (HDL) to fight heart disease. In Spanish studies, rats fed olive oil showed a lower risk for colon cancer. Olive oil lubricates your system, which makes everything work better. It activates the natural production of bile secretions and pancreatic hormones to strengthen digestion, relieve gastritis, and help prevent gallstones, and it strengthens the liver and spleen. Topically, olive oil moisturizes the skin, helps to heal burns and wounds, and prevents the spread of skin eruptions. It's also an excellent scalp conditioner to promote healthy hair.

Types of Olive Oil

EXTRA VIRGIN: The only way to guarantee that your olive oil is pure is to choose extra virgin olive oil. Extra virgin is the oil that comes from the first press of the olives, which yields the purest oil, the truest aroma of olive, and the highest concentration of vitamins, minerals, and antioxidants. To achieve extra virgin status on its label, the olive oil must be cold pressed, without heat, closest to its natural state, free of chemicals, additives, or off flavors.

VIRGIN: The oil comes from the second press of the olives. It's less potent.

PURE: Not pure, in the strict sense of the word, it's processed, filtered, and refined, and can be a combination of a small amount of extra virgin olive oil and a refined olive oil.

LIGHT: A term that may relate to the oil's light color, but *light* is not an official classification for olive oils; therefore, there is no guarantee of its contents, which can include other vegetable oils.

EXTRA LIGHT: This is a highly processed oil with only a trace of true olive flavor.

Four Essentials at Their Best

Let's take a moment to glance back at the first four vital essentials to enhance your health. They are all you need to make two great recipes:

Lemon Garlic Oil

> 2 teaspoons fresh lemon juice
> 2 cloves fresh garlic, mashed
> ⅓ cup extra virgin olive oil

Preparation. Combine ingredients and blend.

Parsley Puree

> 1 cup fresh parsley
> 2 teaspoons fresh lemon juice
> 2 cloves fresh garlic
> ⅓ cup extra virgin olive oil

Preparation. Combine ingredients in a chopper and mince.

Lemon Garlic Oil makes an excellent sauté for vegetables and meats. Drizzle it into a pita or spoon it over a green salad for a rich dressing, and use it in baked casseroles to enrich their flavor.

Parsley Puree makes an excellent sauté, stuffing, or topping for chicken and fish, and can be used as filling for a pita, topped with sliced tomatoes and Parmesan. If you can't eat garlic, use two teaspoons of chopped leeks as a substitute for garlic. Their health virtues are similar to those of garlic and they have a very mellow flavor.

You have four vital essentials to enhance your immunity, protect your heart, strengthen your digestion, fight fatigue and premature aging—but that's not all! You also have two fabulous recipes with lots of versatility! Could it get any easier to guard your most precious possession—your health?

CHAPTER 6

Herbs and Spices for Butter, Honey, and Salt

Think of the pleasure you can discover when you open your refrigerator and find a gourmet assortment of herbal spreads. Never again, the same taste in vegetables, potatoes, and sautés. Never again, the same toast or bagel. You can have thyme toast one day, a poppy seed bagel with lemon-parsley spread on the following day, sage spread on baked oven bread for dinner the next day.

We all have our favorite when it comes to spreads. Years ago, when I wanted to reduce the fat content in my diet, like many people, I switched from butter to margarine. I found that margarine didn't have a harmonious nature for cooking, as butter did, but I stayed with it for the lower fat content, using butter now and then for a treat. Then concerns surfaced about the hydrogenated fats in margarine and their ability to raise levels of bad cholesterol (HDL), so I switched to an olive oil spread (Olivio), which has no hydrogenated fats, a rich flavor, and a smooth texture for cooking. It also includes whey, a healthy source of protein, and olive oil, which lowers bad cholesterol.

Note: For your convenience in *The Magic Teaspoon*, I'll refer to all spreads—butter, margarine, and olive oil spread—as *butter*, and you can use your preferred spread.

When it comes to spreads, whether yours is butter, margarine, or an olive oil spread, you can give them a big boost in pleasure and health in one simple step: herbalize them.

One pound of butter can become four fabulous herbal spreads in minutes! Store them in small refrigerator bowls decorated with an herbal design for a gourmet touch to charm every day. They're easy to make and so delectable, your taste buds will crave the refreshing flavor and lighter feeling you get with herbal energy in your spread. Wake up your menu in a snap, and reap the health benefits of the herbs at the same time!

EZ Herbal Spreads

Use one stick or one cup of butter (one tub in a four-tub pack) for each herbal spread.

Fresh herbs provide the most vivid flavor in spreads, but they are not always available or convenient for most people. If you use dried herbs, keep in mind that dried herbs are more densely packed than fresh herbs; therefore, they are more potent.

Use this simple two-for-one formula for using fresh or dried herbs in any recipe: two teaspoons fresh herbs equals one teaspoon dried herbs.

The following recipe is for parsley butter, but you can use sage, thyme, garlic, or your favorite herb in place of parsley. Only three ingredients!

🌿 *Herbal Butter Recipe*

1 stick *or* 1 cup of butter (use stick butter at room temperature)
1 tablespoon fresh lemon juice
4 teaspoons fresh parsley, minced (or 2 teaspoons dried parsley)

Preparation. Using a blender or whisk, cream the butter, while gradually adding the lemon juice. Blend in parsley and chill.

That's all there is to it! Your everyday butter is enhanced with an antioxidant, blood builder, cancer fighter, and green energizer—parsley.

Gourmet Favorites

- *Thyme Spread.* Replace parsley with 4 teaspoons fresh thyme, minced (or 2 teaspoons dried thyme, crushed).

- *Garlic Spread.* Use 2 fresh garlic cloves, crushed or minced, to replace parsley. To crush garlic cloves, take a large knife, lay the flat blade (near the handle) on the garlic cloves, and press down hard. You can also use a mortar and pestle to crush garlic.

- *Lemon-Sage Spread.* Use sage to replace parsley and add ½ teaspoon shredded lemon peel for extra zest.

- *Lemon-Parsley Spread.* Add ¼ teaspoon shredded lemon peel to the parsley blend for an ultralemony flavor.

- *Toasted Poppy Seed Spread.* Lightly toast 2 teaspoons of poppy seeds in a frying pan to burst their flavor. Use them to replace parsley. It's a fantastic spread for egg noodles, angel hair pasta, and many vegetables.

- *Chive Spread.* Replace parsley with 4 teaspoons fresh minced chives (or 2 teaspoons dried chives, crushed).

Feeling adventurous? Make fresh butter for your herbal spread! Only two ingredients:

✌ *Fresh Butter Recipe*

1 cup of heavy cream
½ cup of ice water

Preparation. In a covered blender on high speed, whip the cream until it settles into a spin at the bottom of the blender. Remove the cover while the cream is spinning to let the air penetrate the blend, and continue at high speed until the cream is whipped. Add the ice water, cover again, and continue to blend on high speed. Watch the butter form in one or two minutes. Use a sieve to drain the butter, add salt to the butter, or lemon pepper for zest, and chill.

Energize Your Honey
for Health and Pleasure

Called bottled sunshine, honey is nectar from flowers—natural fruit sugars that absorb slowly to provide energy over a long term for endurance. Honey has a more stable effect on your blood sugar than does white sugar. Honey is antibacterial to fight infections, it helps to speed healing and recovery, and it contains antioxidants and micro-nutrients, which include citric and amino acids, enzyme, B-complex, folic acid, vitamin C, magnesium, calcium, sodium, silicon, chlorine, copper, sulfur, and iron. Honey is sweeter than sugar, so a little goes a long way. Boost the flavor and energize your honey with herbs and spices!

One jar of honey can become four jars of herb or spice honey. Herb and spice honeys are rich, delicious, and easy to make. They add a wide range of flavors to the sweetness of honey to bring extra pleasure and healing power to your menu every time your use them. Collect four small jelly jars or buy four small glass jars with airtight tops.

❧ *Herbal Honey Recipe*

½ cup honey
4 teaspoons fresh herb or spice (or 2 teaspoons dried)

Preparation. Combine honey with an herb or spice in a jar, cover the jar, and place it in a small amount of gently boiling water. Simmer 30 minutes. Remove the jar from the water and cool. Store it in a cool, dark place for one week before using.

Should You Use Fresh or Dried Herbs for Herbal Honey?

Traditionally, herbal honey has been made with fresh herbs, but fresh herbs are not always convenient for most people. I made my honeys with dried herbs to test the effect, since dried herbs are the most common form of herbs that most people use. One of my goals in *The Magic Teaspoon* is to make complicated things easier and more realistic for the average person, who loves pleasure but also loves convenience (like me). Fresh herbal honey is exquisite, but I found that dried herbs produced rich and delicious honeys that I really enjoy, and the convenience is a very important asset. If you use dried herbs, crush them and grind them with a pestle to a more powdery texture before you add them to the honey to break their bonds and enhance the flavor.

After you make your herbal honey, if you find that the honey is too herbal for you, simply add more honey and blend it in. If you find that the honey is not as herbal as you'd like, add more herb and heat it again.

✺ *Spice Honey Recipe*

½ cup honey
2 teaspoons fresh or powdered spice

Preparation. See instructions for Herbal Honey. In the case of spices, which are already dried, use the same amount whether dried or powdered when you are making honey with spices. Begin with 2 teaspoons and experiment with the taste until you reach the potency you desire. Break whole seeds with a pestle and grind them down into powder. Chapter 2, "Nature's Bouquet of Healing Herbs and Spices for Cooking," will give you specific instructions on how to use the whole seeds of each spice.

Ten minutes from now, you can have four herb or spice honeys simmering in your kitchen. Choose herbs or spices for your honey based on the health benefits you would like to receive—see "Nature's Bouquet of Healing Herbs and Spices for Cooking" to make your choices—or you can make herbal honeys just for pleasure and receive the health benefits as a bonus. The aromatic herbs, flowers, and rich green herbs make excellent honey. I routinely make four honeys from dried herbs and spices that I love. My four favorite honeys are:

- *Fennel Honey.* Fennel has a soothing nature, and it's a marvelous herb for digestive strength. I use good quality dried, powdered fennel to make my honey. It's available in a shaker in natural food grocery stores that carry herbs and spices.

- *Coriander Spice Honey.* This is my nectar. It lifts my spirits instantly, and it's a real energizer.

- *Thyme Honey.* When bees dine on thyme, the honey they produce is considered one of the richest in the world. Thyme is also one of the best herbs to fight infections, particularly in your respiratory system.

- *Rosemary Honey.* Rosemary gives honey a rich, piney taste. It stimulates circulation, enhances memory, and it's good for your heart.

Other honeys to try:

- *Spearmint Honey.* A minty defense against colds, flu, and infections.

- *Calendula (Marigold) Honey.* A lymph-cleansing honey, important for women, to keep the lymph system free of infections, since the lymph system plays a role in breast cancer.

- *Chive Flower Honey.* A body tonic and blood builder for vitality.

- *Anise Honey.* A natural anti-inflammatory and time-honored honey for respiratory strength and to fight emphysema.

The possibilities for health-enriching honeys are limitless. Let yourself have fun with your experiment in making herbal honey. When you find special herb or spice honeys that you love, spread your pleasure by giving a small jar or a selection of jars to your friends. Put your name on the label—after all, you made it yourself.

Salt from the Sea

Sea salt is made from naturally evaporated seawater. Seawater, in its original state, has more than eighty minerals and trace elements that support the nerves, glands, and brain activity, and it is well known that natural salt baths can have a healing effect on the body. Sodium from seawater is easier for the body to assimilate than standard table salt, which means less stress on your system. Sea salt also contains iodine and some trace minerals it retains from the sea. It has a fresh taste, and a little goes a long way for cooking and table use. It also comes in an iodized version.

Standard table salt is less balanced: it is approximately 60 percent chloride and 40 percent sodium, with added flowing agents, and it lacks the natural minerals and trace elements that sea salt can retain.

Use salt sparingly, since excess salt creates stress on the kidneys, and it can inhibit your natural circulation, causing migraines. Your heart has to work too hard when there is too much salt in your system.

Make Your Own Herb and Spice Salter

One hidden benefit of herbs and spices in your everyday menu is the effect they have on your taste buds. They enhance the flavor of your food, making salt seem less mandatory as a seasoning. A combination of herbs and spices as a salter can go a long way to minimize the desire for salt and help you curtail your salt intake.

Make your own herb and spice salter without using sodium. Combine your favorite herbs and spices to suit your taste. Don't worry about making mistakes. The way to find your own perfect blend is to experiment, and the reduction you'll see in your salt intake is well worth the effort. For your herb and spice salter, choose dried herbs that don't have added salt. For instance, garlic comes in two shaker versions, garlic powder (only the dried herb) and garlic salt. Your best choice is the true herb, garlic powder. This gives you control over your salt intake instead of finding it in an herbal shaker as a surprise.

Try this blend of herbs and spices for your salter. It enhances the taste of food, instead of simply salting it.

✿ Rev It Up

Five great herbs and spices combine in Rev It Up to give you a full body tonic, a circulatory stimulant, and a potent infection fighter, with a soothing effect on your nerves to fight anxiety.

    4 teaspoons dried parsley
    4 teaspoons dried dill
    2 teaspoons dried mustard powder
    1 teaspoon dried or ground garlic*
    1 teaspoon cayenne pepper

*Garlic also comes ground, which has a fresher taste than garlic powder. If you can't find ground garlic, use garlic powder, but not garlic salt.

Preparation. Combine ingredients and blend. Transfer the blend to a salt shaker and shake it routinely to keep the powdery herbs and spices from settling on the bottom. If you would like a larger quantity, use this ratio: 1 cup parsley, 1 cup dill, ½ cup mustard, ¼ cup garlic, and ¼ cup cayenne.

Celery Seed Salter

A natural salt substitute is celery seeds, which come in commercial shakers. Celery seeds have a salty taste and can be a valuable aid for people on a salt-restricted diet or for those who can't eat onions. Celery seeds are also a natural antacid and antiseptic to cleanse the bladder and fight urinary tract infections. They help to remove uric acid from the kidneys and stimulate blood flow to flush wastes from muscles and joints, which is beneficial for arthritis. Chinese studies show that celery lowers blood pressure, and the seeds are rich in potassium, sodium, calcium, iron, silicon, and vitamins A, B-complex, and C. Be sure to check the label to guarantee that you are getting celery seeds alone, not celery salt.

YOUR OWN MORTAR AND PESTLE

A mortar and pestle has come to symbolize herbalists, dating back to times when herbs and spices were the only medicines, but it is much more than a symbol. Cooking with herbs and spices is so much easier when you have a mortar and pestle. You can crush seeds, nuts, and dried herbs in a flash. Many herbs and spices, such as dried rosemary, thyme, and aniseed can have a sticklike texture, and it's a good idea to crush them before you use them. It breaks their bonds and releases a fuller aroma. You can crush larger dried herbs like chives into smaller pieces to get a more harmonious blend. There are myriad uses for a mortar and pestle in a modern kitchen. I use mine to crush those big, hard vitamins that can't be swallowed with ease, and I mix the vitamin powder into Natural Applesauce (see the recipe in the next chapter). That way, I can swallow them with ease, and vitamins digest more naturally when you take them along with food.

When I was the managing editor of a medical magazine based in Boston, the doctor who was the founder of the magazine had an antique white stone mortar and pestle on his desk, which he had kept from his early days in medical school. In those days, I admired the mortar and pestle as an antique. These days, I admire it as a modern kitchen essential.

CHAPTER 7

Breakfast Energy

Breakfast is the most vital meal of the day to boost your health and fuel the flame of your metabolism. While you are sleeping, your body downshifts into a resting state, which slows down your digestion and burns calories at a greatly reduced rate. The only way to bring your body out of this reduced metabolic state is by giving it high-energy food. Without that early morning nutrition, you are forcing your body to work on stress rather than nutrients for the first valuable hours in the day.

Dieters who skip breakfast are making a mistake. Your body will continue to burn calories at a greatly reduced rate all morning if you don't eat breakfast, and you'll lose weight more slowly. You'll notice the difference in stamina and health when you eat an energizing breakfast. Good food is a gift of pleasure you can give yourself every morning to start your day in the right spirit.

Feature: Muffin Heaven

Muffin lovers will delight in these unique muffin recipes. Make them in the evening, freeze half, and use the rest for breakfast treats.

🌿 Jalapeño Corn Muffins

This is a corn muffin to wake up your senses. Men seem to have a special taste for them. You can make this recipe half-and-half—half with jalapeño and half without—for a bonus! Great corn muffins and jalapeño muffins from one recipe. Low in sugar and rich in taste. Makes 10–12 muffins.

1 cup fine cornmeal
¼ cup coarse cornmeal
1 cup flour (or spelt flour for wheat-sensitive people)
⅓ cup sugar
3 teaspoons baking powder
1 teaspoon baking soda
½ teaspoon salt
1 cup canned corn niblets, drained
1 cup milk
1 tablespoon vinegar
1 egg
¼ cup butter, softened
½ cup jalapeño pepper, chopped

Preparation. Preheat oven to 400 degrees. Grease muffin pans with butter. Set out 2 bowls. In bowl 1, combine cornmeal, flour, sugar, baking powder, baking soda, and salt. Blend. Add corn niblets and blend. In bowl 2, combine milk and vinegar; stir. Add egg and butter, and beat with whisk. Combine bowls 1 and 2 and blend. Add jalapeño and stir. Pour into muffin pans. Bake 15–20 minutes.

🌿 *Spicy Pear Muffins*

Three great spices give this muffin its exotic flavor—vanilla, nutmeg, and ginger—with lots of healing power, including antioxidants. Makes 8 large muffins or a dozen small.

2 large pears, peeled, cored and diced	¼ teaspoon salt
½ cup sugar	½ teaspoon ginger
¼ cup vegetable oil	½ teaspoon nutmeg
1 large egg, beaten	1 cup flour
1 teaspoon vanilla	½ cup chopped pecans
1 teaspoon baking soda	½ cup raisins or dates (golden raisins for color harmony)

Preparation. Preheat oven to 325 degrees. Grease 8 muffin cups. Set out 2 bowls. In bowl 1, combine pears and sugar. In bowl 2, blend vegetable oil, egg, and vanilla. Combine bowls 1 and 2. Add baking soda, salt, ginger, and nutmeg. Stir well. Add flour and mix gently. Fold in nuts and raisins. Spoon batter into muffin cups. Bake 30 minutes.

🌿 *Muffin and Herbal Butter*

Top your muffin with herbal butter for a boost of energy. Try these combinations:

Chive butter on your plain corn muffin

Tarragon butter on your Jalapeño Corn Muffin

Warm ginger butter on your Spicy Pear Muffin. Use grated fresh ginger—½ teaspoon of ginger to 2 teaspoons of butter in a saucepan—warm, and blend.

🌿 *Muffin and Spice*

Blend a spice into yogurt for a zesty topping with extra health benefits.

    ¼ cup plain yogurt
    ½ teaspoon cinnamon or nutmeg

🌿 *Natural Applesauce*

Make your own applesauce for a healthy fruit topping on your muffin. You'll get a significant reduction in sugar from that found in processed applesauce. Natural Applesauce is a cinch to make, and you can even use apples that are going soft. The trick is, don't think you have to make a whole jar. You can also use this applesauce as a fruit snack on its own or as a fruit with lunch or dinner. For an ultrarich Natural Applesauce topping, blend the applesauce with yogurt and chopped walnuts.

    3 sweet red apples, cored and diced
    ⅓ cup water
    ¼ teaspoon cinnamon

Preparation. Cut a few sweet red apples in chunks, remove the cores but retain the skins, and chop them into small pieces in a food processor or blender. Put them in a saucepan with water and cinnamon on low simmer. As the apples break down, break them into smaller chunks. Keep an eye on the water level while they are cooking to insure that the apples aren't sticking to the pan. When you are pleased with the consistency, remove them from the heat—8–10 minutes. Serve warm, or chill in a small jar.

🌿 *Fancy Muffin*

For a special treat, top your muffin with the works!

  ½ cup of fresh fruit, diced
  Dollop of dessert whip
  Dash of cinnamon and a cherry on top

🌿 *Thyme Toast and Fried Eggs*

Have an aromatic morning with thyme on your toast, eggs for protein, and invigorating parsley as a garnish. You'll boost your immunity and set yourself up for a healthy day.

  1 teaspoon crushed thyme (or 2 teaspoons fresh)
  2 teaspoons butter
  2 slices toast
  2 fried eggs
  1 teaspoon chopped fresh parsley

Preparation. Crush dried thyme or chop fresh thyme. Spread butter on toast and sprinkle equal portions of thyme on each slice. Use a toaster oven or regular oven (with toast on an open rack to toast both sides) and bake at 350 degrees. Toasts in about 1 minute. Serve 2 fried eggs on the side, garnished with 1 teaspoon fresh chopped parsley.

❧ Oatmeal with Cinnamon and Golden Raisins

Cinnamon is a circulatory tonic to give your body a boost in the morning, and it helps to reduce your blood sugar level. Oats have a natural antibiotic and lots of nutrition, and they help to reduce your cholesterol.

> 1 cup of hot oatmeal cereal
> ½ teaspoon cinnamon
> ¼ cup golden raisins (or chopped almonds, for sugar-restricted diets)

Preparation. Cook oatmeal according to package instructions. Just as it comes off the heat, blend in cinnamon and raisins. Also try oatmeal with cinnamon, honey, and walnuts.

❧ Bulgur Cereal with Cinnamon, Honey, and Almonds

Bulgur is the wheat used in tabouli; it has a rich, nutty taste. Honey gives bulgur a lingering sweetness and energy to start the day pampered with pleasure. It leaves you feeling satisfied for hours.

> 1 cup bulgur wheat
> 1 teaspoon cinnamon
> 2 teaspoons honey
> ¼ cup chopped almonds

Preparation. Bulgar comes in instant and standard versions. Follow package directions to make. Blend in cinnamon, honey, and almonds just as it comes off the heat. Also try bulgur with cinnamon and golden raisins.

⚘ *Fantastic Fried Eggs*

Something special for your morning! These eggs have a sweet, refreshing taste and rich herbal energy that contents you for hours. Try it! You'll be amazed.

    1 clove garlic
    1 teaspoon butter or olive oil
    2 eggs
    2 teaspoons fresh parsley, minced (or 1 teaspoon dried)
    Salt and pepper to taste

Preparation. Sauté garlic in butter or olive oil. Break the eggs over the garlic. Just before you flip the eggs, sprinkle fresh minced parsley leaves over the top of the eggs. Salt and pepper and serve.

⚘ *Tangy Tarragon Omelet*

A lush flavor with a sweet nature. If you can't find fresh tarragon leaves, use dried, but try to use fresh parsley. Serves 2.

    Herbal Filling
    ½ cup yellow pepper, diced
    ½ cup mushrooms, diced
    2 teaspoons fresh parsley, chopped (or 1 teaspoon dried)
    2 teaspoons fresh tarragon (or 1 teaspoon dried)
    1 teaspoon olive oil

    1 clove garlic, diced
    1 teaspoon butter
    4 eggs, beaten with a dash of water
    Optional: 2 slices white cheese (Swiss, goat, American)

Preparation. Sauté first four Herbal Filling ingredients in 1 teaspoon of olive oil; set aside. To make omelet, sauté garlic in butter. Add eggs. When eggs set, add Herbal Filling, top with cheese, and fold.

✿ Tex-Mex Omelet with Sauce

Omelets are a fabulous way to get lots of vegetable and herbal energy in one dish. Have a zesty morning! Serves 2.

Herbal Filling
1 cup mushrooms, diced
½ cup red onion, diced
2 cloves garlic, diced
2 jalapeño peppers, minced
1 cup fresh cilantro, chopped (or parsley)
1 teaspoon olive oil

4 eggs, beaten with a dash of water
1 teaspoon butter

Preparation. In food processor or chopper, chop first five Herbal Filling ingredients, and sauté in 1 teaspoon olive oil. Set aside. Cook eggs in 1 teaspoon butter. When eggs are set, add Herbal Filling just before folding. Smother with Tex-Mex sauce.

Tex-Mex Sauce
4 plum tomatoes, with juice, diced (or 1 small can)
1 teaspoon dried coriander
3 teaspoons fresh lime juice
Dash of olive oil
Salt and pepper to taste

Preparation. Combine ingredients, simmer, and stir to blend. Spoon over omelet.

🌿 One Great Omelet for Herbal Versatility with Magic Teaspoon Purees

Use the following omelet recipe as a standard, and charm it with your choice of an herbal puree from chapter 8. Omelets made this way—with vegetables, herbs, and protein from eggs—are an all-in-one dish! They make great dinners, too. The puree can be used as filling or topping. Try it first as a topping. Serves 2.

Herbal Filling
½ cup mushrooms, diced
½ cup onion, diced
2 cloves garlic, diced
1 teaspoon olive oil

4 eggs, beaten with a dash of water
1 teaspoon butter

Preparation. Sauté first three Herbal Filling ingredients in 1 teaspoon olive oil. Set aside. Cook eggs in 1 teaspoon butter, and add Herbal Filling just before folding. Top with a puree (see chapter 8) for pure pleasure and powerful energy.

BASIL BLISS OMELET. Sweet-natured basil makes this omelet's character lushly Italian. Add 4 teaspoons of Basil Bliss (see chapter 8) to ½ cup of cottage cheese, and spin it in a chopper or blender. Spoon it over the omelet.

GARLIC WHAMMO OMELET. Garlic lovers will delight in this rich puree as a topping or filling. It's a burst of energy you feel instantly. Add 4 teaspoons of Garlic Whammo (see chapter 8) to ½ cup of cottage cheese, and spin it in a chopper or blender. Fill your omelet or spoon it over the top.

DILL DELIVERANCE OMELET. This piney green puree is one of the best nerve tonics in the herbal kingdom. It has a soothing nature, but it delivers lots of energy, too, and it's a blood builder. For a change of pace, combine 4 teaspoons of Dill Deliverance (see chapter 8) with ½ cup of sour cream, and spin it in a chopper or blender. Spoon it over your omelet.

🌿 Scrambled Eggs

This exquisite recipe can become several different versions of scrambled eggs. A hint of onion and garlic highlight the flavor of scrambled eggs like nothing else can. The filling is one herb and one cheese of your choice. This recipe is based on one serving, so you can get the gist of it easily.

> 1 tablespoon onion, finely chopped
> ½ clove garlic, finely chopped
> 1 teaspoon butter
> 2 eggs with 2 teaspoons water (1 teaspoon per egg)

Preparation. Sauté onion and garlic in butter until onion is transparent. Beat eggs with water. Now:

Choose 1 herb: Add ½ teaspoon dried or 1 teaspoon fresh herb to beaten eggs. Use tarragon, dill, parsley, basil, or chives. You can combine 2 herbs, but keep the total quantity to ½ teaspoon dried or 1 teaspoon fresh herb. This recipe relies on subtlety.

Choose 1 cheese: Crumble 2 tablespoons cheese to add to eggs when they have set in the pan. Use crumbled goat cheese, crumbled Gorgonzola, crumbled blue cheese. Scramble and Enjoy!

Think of the possibilities—dill and goat cheese, tarragon and blue cheese, parsley and Gorgonzola, basil and blue cheese, chives and Gorgonzola . . . on and on into herbal paradise. Delicate and light. Try them all!

BREAKFAST BUFFET IN YOUR FRIDGE

If you're on the run and don't have time to prepare breakfast, store these breakfast items in a large, flat refrigerator box to insure that you and your kids have a nourishing breakfast readily available every day. Simply reach in and pull out the box to make a healthy breakfast in a jiffy. Close the lid and return the rest to the fridge. Refurbish every few days. For company (if you have to leave early for work), tack a note to the fridge telling your guests to look inside the breakfast buffet box, and leave a saucepan on the stove for eggs.

Selection of muffins
Herbal butters in small jars
Toppings in small jars (yogurt, herbal honey, or Natural Applesauce)
Container of sliced fruits
Measured portions for 1 cup of cereal in ziplock bags
Ziplock bags with nuts
Ziplock bags or small boxes of raisins (golden and regular)
Fresh eggs in a container, or hard-boiled eggs, peeled, in a ziplock bag

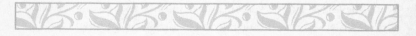

CHAPTER 8

High-Energy, High-Potency Herbal Purees

You Won't Know How You Lived Without Them

These potent herbal purees are instant energizers! They wake up your senses and give you rich health benefits! They also make high-energy eating easy and versatile! This is the way to eat for power, pleasure, and satisfaction. When you make a puree, store the potent blend in a glass jar in your refrigerator; it will retain its freshness for two weeks. You can use teaspoons of each puree in a variety of ways:

- as an herbal base for sauces and gravies

- as an herbal booster for pasta sauces

- as an herbal blend to energize burgers, rice dishes, and stir fry sauces

- as a stuffing or basting for chicken or fish

- blended with butter for an herbal spread on oven-baked breads

- Best of all, make a creamy puree blend with cottage cheese, sour cream, yogurt, or yogurt cheese. You get an instant dip for vegetables; a topping for meats, fish, rice, pasta, and beans; a sandwich filling; or an herbal spread for toast or crackers. The versatility of these purees is as wide as your imagination. I use dollops of the creamy puree blends on every lunch and dinner plate, just for pleasure. You'll find the recipes for the creamy puree blends after the recipes for the purees.

Bonus for Dieters

These herbal purees have such a rich taste, you can use low-fat versions of cottage cheese, sour cream, and yogurt for your blends, and you won't even know they're the low-fat versions. They give you instant pleasure and satisfaction with rich herbal energy! Keep a variety of creamy puree blends in your refrigerator for snacks and to satisfy hunger pangs, and never feel deprived on a diet again!

Garlic Whammo

A flecked, forest-green puree that turns bright minty green when you blend it into cottage cheese, sour cream, or yogurt. Its nature is pure energy and healing power.

    2 cups fresh parsley, stems removed
    6–8 small cloves garlic, chopped
    ½ cup green pepper, chopped
    ⅓ cup olive oil

Preparation. Combine all ingredients in a food processor, chopper, or blender, and blend to an even consistency. Once or twice, turn the machine off and scrape the sides of the bowl to resettle the ingredients on the bottom. Refrigerate half of the puree plain, and blend the rest into cottage cheese, sour cream, or yogurt. Chill it for one hour to have an energizing dip or spread ready for snacking.

℀ Dill Deliverance

This piney green puree has a fragrance that is enchanting. Its nature is soothing and uplifting, and it fights depression. I make the puree without garlic to maintain its mellow nature, but garlic lovers can add two or three cloves of garlic to the blend.

- ½ large package fresh spinach (or 1 package frozen, cooked and drained)
- ½ cup fresh dill, chopped (or 4–6 teaspoons dried dill)
- ⅓ cup olive oil
- 1 teaspoon chile powder

Preparation. Combine all ingredients in a food processor, chopper, or blender, and blend to an even consistency. Once or twice, turn the machine off and scrape the sides of the bowl to resettle the ingredients on the bottom. Refrigerate half of the puree plain, and blend the rest into cottage cheese, sour cream, or yogurt. Chill it for one hour to have an instant high-energy dip ready for snacking.

🌿 *Basil Bliss*

A sweet, rich, green puree that lifts your spirit and gives you greater immune system strength.

> 2 cups fresh parsley, stems removed
> 1 cup fresh basil leaves, chopped
> 4 small cloves of garlic, chopped
> ½ cup green pepper, chopped
> ⅓ cup olive oil

Preparation. Chop all ingredients in a food processor, chopper, or blender, and blend to an even consistency. Once or twice, turn the machine off and scrape the sides of the bowl to resettle the ingredients on the bottom. Refrigerate half of the puree plain, and blend the rest into cottage cheese, sour cream, or yogurt. Chill it for one hour to have an instant high-energy dip or spread ready for snacking.

🌿 *Basil Bliss with Dried Basil*

Dried basil cannot equal the taste of fresh basil in a puree; however, you can come very close with this method for making Basil Bliss with dried basil. I tested it on several friends, and they couldn't tell the difference between the fresh basil puree and the dried basil puree. This recipe is for everyone who forgets to freeze fresh basil for winter.

Preparation. Crush ½ cup of good quality dried basil with a mortar and pestle. Soak the crushed basil in 4 teaspoons of olive oil with a dash of lime, a dash of lemon, and a dash of lemon pepper for ten minutes. Crush it again after it has soaked. Add it to the Basil Bliss recipe above as the basil.

🌿 *Roasted Red Pepper Puree*

This puree is delightful plain, as a fresh pepper topping for any dish. The puree below is spiced up to give it a deep, penetrating Asian flavor.

4 large red peppers
2 teaspoons olive oil

Spice Blend
1 teaspoon aniseed, crushed
½ teaspoon cinnamon
½ teaspoon ginger
½ teaspoon allspice

Preparation. Preheat oven to 350 degrees and place peppers in a baking dish. Roast 10–15 minutes, or until skin is blackened, or peppers collapse when pressed. Cool. Peel off skin and combine roasted peppers with 2 teaspoons olive oil in a food processor or chopper, and blend to an even consistency. Use additional olive oil if needed to achieve a smooth blend. Make the spice blend separately in a small bowl, add ¾ to the puree, and taste; add the remaining spice blend gradually to suit your taste. I like it deep and spicy, so I add the whole amount. (See chapter 10, "Sumptuous Salads and Fresh Salad Dressings," for Roasted Red Pepper Vinaigrette salad dressing).

Creamy Puree Blends

COTTAGE CHEESE BLEND. Combine 4 teaspoons of an herbal puree in ½ to 1 cup of cottage cheese, and spin it in a chopper or blender until you reach a creamy consistency. This is a high-charged herbal delight with a low-fat attitude. Spread it on crackers, use it as a filling for sandwiches, or dollop it on green salads, vegetables, toast, muffins, bagels, and oven-baked bread. I eat it for a snack when I need energy.

SOUR CREAM OR YOGURT BLEND. Combine 4 teaspoons of an herbal puree in ½ cup of sour cream, and spin it in a chopper or blender until you reach a creamy consistency. This is mellow herbal magic. Dollop it on soups and beans, use it for dips, paint it over chicken cutlets or fish, or lick it off the spoon while you make the puree—you won't be able to resist.

CREAM CHEESE PUREE. Combine 4 teaspoons of an herbal puree in ½ to 1 cup of cream cheese, and spin it in a chopper or blender until you reach a creamy consistency. Since cream cheese is denser than cottage cheese or sour cream, if you want it creamier, add a dash of olive oil to thin out the blend. This is seventh heaven. Use it to top or fill omelets, spread it on a sandwich, combine it with chopped nuts for dips, and let yourself dream about the possibilities.

Creamy Yogurt Cheese Blend

A superior cheese to give you the health benefits of yogurt with the texture of cream cheese. It's plain yogurt with the moisture removed, leaving you with a ball of thick yogurt cheese.

Make Your Own Yogurt Cheese

Yogurt cheese is so easy to make, and so much fun when you see the results. You're going to take the moisture out of a quart of plain yogurt. You need only a package of cheesecloth (try your local hardware store) and a quart of plain yogurt. Full-fat yogurt is best, low fat is acceptable, but fat-free won't give you the creamy consistency you want in this cheese.

STEP 1: Add ⅛ teaspoon sea salt to the quart of yogurt, and blend. Empty the yogurt into a long piece of cheesecloth. Knot it once, right next to the yogurt, and tie the free ends to one of the bars on a shelf in your refrigerator. Place a bowl directly under the yogurt, on the shelf below.

STEP 2: Go to bed and have a good night's sleep. The moisture will drain from the yogurt into the bowl while you sleep, and when you open the cheesecloth the next morning—eureka! It's yogurt cheese. It's ready for anything.

If you don't have cheesecloth, try this modern method: Line a colander with a stand with two paper towels, pour the yogurt in, set the colander in a bowl to catch the water from the yogurt, and cover the top of the colander with plastic wrap. Leave it overnight in your refrigerator. If you find that the yogurt cheese isn't thoroughly dry in the morning, wrap it in dry paper towels and squeeze out excess moisture. The best modern method might be a combination—line the colander with cheesecloth, which you can lift out of the colander, wrap around the cheese, and tighten at the top to squeeze excess moisture out.

Dress yogurt cheese with your favorite herbs to use as an herbal cheese snack; a spread or topping for sandwiches, crackers, beans, omelets, and baked bread; or a filling or topping for any main dish. Use this formula to make yogurt cheese into an herbal topping or spread:

½ cup yogurt cheese
1 teaspoon olive oil
1 teaspoon fresh lemon juice
Dash of white pepper (for color harmony)
½ cup fresh herb (or herbs), chopped (or ¼ cup dried herbs)

❧ *Parsley and Garlic Yogurt Cheese Spread*

½ cup yogurt cheese
1 teaspoon olive oil
1 teaspoon fresh lemon juice
Dash of white pepper
½ cup fresh parsley, chopped
2 cloves garlic, minced

Preparation. Combine ingredients and blend. If you want a creamier spread, add olive oil gradually until you reach the consistency you desire. Store the spread in the refrigerator to be ready for any sandwich.

❧ *Dill Deliverance* Yogurt Cheese Spread*

4 teaspoons Dill Deliverance puree
½ cup yogurt cheese
1 teaspoon lemon juice
Dash of white pepper to taste

Preparation. Combine ingredients and blend. Store in the refrigerator to be ready for any sandwich.

*Use Garlic Whammo, Basil Bliss, or Roasted Red Pepper Puree in the same ratio. The purees already contain olive oil, so wait to add olive oil until you gauge the consistency. Use additional olive oil to reach the consistency you desire.

❦ *Fried Yogurt Cheese Patty in a Pita*

Use Yogurt Cheese plain or herbed, and form a patty. Fry the patty in a skillet with a dash of olive oil (and I mean a dash) until each side is light brown. If it crumbles in the pan, you used too much olive oil, but don't fret. I like yogurt cheese crumbled in a pita, so I intentionally crumble the patty in the pan and spoon it into the pita. Drizzle a dash of olive oil in a pita, line the sides with sliced tomatoes, and add the yogurt patty or crumbled yogurt cheese. It's utterly delicious. The taste is so refreshing, you'll start to crave it, and you can use your favorite herbs to vary the flavor. Consider a garnish of sliced olives for your next cheese patty pita. Experiment with the possibilities. It never gets boring.

❦ *Yogurt Cheese–Mint Pita Grilled*

This is a classic Lebanese blend to combine with yogurt cheese. It's ultraminty and so refreshing, you'll think you're lunching on the Mediterranean in summer.

- ½ cup yogurt cheese
- 1 teaspoon olive oil
- 1 teaspoon lemon juice
- ½ cup fresh mint, chopped

Preparation. Combine the ingredients and blend. Drizzle olive oil in a pita, fill the pita with yogurt cheese blend, and grill the pita under the broiler for a minute. It's also delightful cold with sliced tomatoes.

CHAPTER 9

Sauces and Dips at Your Fingertips

You can transform your everyday meals into a powerful health menu simply by focusing on two main areas of your daily diet: toppings and dips. Keep an assortment of fresh toppings and dips in your refrigerator to feed your hunger urges with high-powered nutrition. They have no sugar, no additives, and such rich tastes that you can use low-fat versions of mayonnaise or sour cream and not even notice.

Also keep fresh cut celery sticks, carrot sticks, red and yellow pepper strips, or your own favorite snacking vegetables in ready-to-eat refrigerator bowls. Don't forget hard-boiled eggs—a fabulous protein snack with an herbal dip. Use toppings and dips to dollop on cooked vegetables, meat, fish, and salads. All the energy you need can be at arm's reach.

Oh yes, you can also eat them with a spoon for a quick energy boost.

Remember to stir any herbal blend that has been refrigerated before you use it, to harmonize the ingredients.

Your key to successful recipes with herbs and spices: **Spice before you salt.**

🌿 *Fresh Salsa*

Deep, rich, red, and zesty! Serves 4, unless you eat it like most people do, by the cup. It makes a great snack with white, unsalted corn chips.

1 large red onion
5 cloves garlic, minced
3 jalapeño chiles, minced
3 tablespoons fresh lime juice
¾ cup chopped fresh cilantro*
1 teaspoon coriander
1–2 teaspoons olive oil
Salt and pepper to taste
2 cans plum tomatoes, seeded, chopped fine

*If you haven't got cilantro, use parsley.

Preparation. Combine all ingredients except tomatoes in a chopper or blender and chop. Chop tomatoes by hand (to avoid mushy effect), add to the other ingredients, and blend gently until fully mixed.

🌿 *Black Bean and Corn Salsa*

Use the Fresh Salsa recipe and add 1 can of black beans (drained) and 1 can of corn (drained).

🌿 *Cool Salsa*

Some like it hot, others do not. For a mellow salsa, use the Fresh Salsa recipe and replace the jalapeño with ½ cup sweet red peppers, chopped.

✌ *Great Green Sauce*

You can make this potent green sauce with spinach or watercress—
and both have great green healing power.

1 cup fresh spinach or watercress, chopped (stems removed)
1 clove garlic, chopped
¼ cup fresh parsley, chopped (stems removed)
2 tablespoons fresh basil leaves (or 1 tablespoon dried)
¼ cup plain yogurt
¼ cup fresh grated Parmesan cheese
½ cup ricotta (or cottage cheese)
Dash of black pepper to taste (fresh or coarsely ground)
½ cup finely chopped onion

Preparation. Combine all ingredients except onion in a chopper or
blender and chop to blend. Add onion to the blend and stir in by
hand.

✌ *Guacamole*

A world favorite. This one is made with parsley and lemon, but you
can vary the flavor by using fresh cilantro instead of parsley and a teaspoon of lime juice instead of lemon.

1 avocado
1–2 cloves garlic, crushed
⅛ teaspoon cayenne
2 tablespoons lemon juice
¼–½ cup Bermuda onion, chopped
2 tablespoons sour cream (*or* mayo *or* yogurt)
1 medium tomato, diced in small chunks

Preparation. Cut avocado in half and scoop out meat. In a blender, combine all ingredients except tomato, which you will fold into the blend by hand to avoid a mushy effect. If you desire a very mellow blend, you can leave out the cayenne and use a dash of salt and pepper instead.

🌿 *Eggplant and Sesame Supreme*

This blend has a rich Middle Eastern mystique. Dollop it on your dinner plate for a treat, spread it in a pita, or use it as a topping for vegetables and meats. Combine it with rice, or blend it into yogurt for a luxurious dip. Try half plain and half with the variation: sage.

   1 medium eggplant
   Juice of 1 lemon
   2 cloves garlic, crushed
   2 teaspoons tahini
   Variation: Add 1 teaspoon dried sage

Preparation. Preheat oven to 450 degrees. Puncture whole eggplant with a fork, and place it on a cookie sheet. Bake for 15 minutes, until very soft. Let cool, remove skin, and place eggplant meat in a food processor or blender with other ingredients. Blend and chill. You can also blend this by hand to achieve a thicker blend; combine the ingredients and mash. If you like very potent blends, add an additional teaspoon of tahini.

✒ *Pesto with Pine Nuts*

This blend is all basil and subtle harmony.

    1 cup fresh basil leaves (press down tightly for measure)
    1 clove garlic, crushed
    1 tablespoon toasted pine nuts
    ¼ cup extra virgin olive oil
    ½ teaspoon salt
    ¼ cup fresh grated Parmesan cheese
    1 tablespoon fresh grated Romano cheese
    1½ tablespoons soft butter
    2 medium tomatoes, peeled and seeded

Preparation. Grind everything except the Parmesan, Romano, butter, and tomatoes in a chopper. Add Parmesan, Romano, butter, and diced tomatoes by hand, and gently blend.

✒ *Pesto with Walnuts*

This blend is deep and potent. Make it with fresh basil leaves only. In the summer, you can stock up on fresh basil, make the pesto in a larger quantity, and freeze it in ice cube trays, covered with clear wrap, to have it available for winter. Remove one or two pesto cubes for use in any pasta or vegetable dish. This recipe will give you a hearty portion.

    1 cup fresh basil leaves, chopped (press down tightly to measure)
    2 large cloves garlic
    ½ cup walnuts, chopped
    ½ cup fresh grated Romano or Parmesan cheese (or ¼ cup of each,
        combined)
    ½ cup olive oil

Preparation. Combine herbs and nuts in food processor, chopper, or blender. Gradually add olive oil to reach an even consistency. Add grated cheese and continue to blend, adding more olive oil, if needed, to smooth the blend.

Feature: Hommus

Hommus means *chickpea* in Arabic. In the Arab world, every family has their own recipe for hommus, and there is no standardized hommus. In Syria, some families make hommus with olive oil, cumin, and allspice instead of tahini and lemon juice. The version that is common in the United States is derived from some of the most famous chickpea preparations from the Levant and Egypt.

Serve Hommus the Traditional Way

Use a large, round serving platter to present hommus to your family and friends. Spoon the hommus onto the platter, and warm 3 tablespoons of extra virgin olive oil. Make fan-shaped furrows in the hommus, and fill the furrows with warm olive oil. Sprinkle toasted pine nuts on top. Garnish the edges with mint leaves, and sprinkle fresh chopped mint on top. Serve with warm Arabic flat bread or pita.

TOASTED PINE NUTS. In small skillet, toast pine nuts in 1 teaspoon olive oil over medium heat until they are light brown (about 4 minutes).

ADDITIONAL GARNISHES. Black olives, pomegranate seeds, cayenne pepper, red Aleppo pepper, ground cumin, or paprika.

CHICKPEAS FOR THE RECIPE. *Raw chickpeas:* If you use raw chickpeas, use 1½ cups of raw chickpeas, and soak them for at least 1½ hours in water. Boil for at least 1½ hours, or until the chickpeas are very soft. *Canned chickpeas:* Canned chickpeas should be removed from the liquid, rinsed, and drained before using. Save the liquid; you can use it to even out the consistency in your blend after you have added the other ingredients.

✿ *Hommus and Cumin*

This recipe uses canned chickpeas, drained and rinsed, for convenience.

2 cups canned chickpeas, drained and rinsed (save the liquid)
3 cloves garlic, minced
3 tablespoons lemon juice
¼ cup water
3 teaspoons tahini
½ teaspoon cumin
½ teaspoon paprika
2 teaspoons olive oil

Preparation. In food processor or chopper*, combine chickpeas, garlic, lemon juice, and water. Process for 1 minute or until smooth. If the blend is too thick, add more water. Stir in tahini, cumin, and paprika. Taste. Adjust flavor with cumin, paprika, lemon, or tahini to preference. If you would like a creamier spread, add liquid from the chickpeas or 1–2 teaspoons olive oil. Chill.

*Note: You can make hommus in a blender but it will take a little longer

Serve Hommus the Modern Way

Spread hommus in shallow bowl and drizzle olive oil over it. Garnish with lemon slices and minced parsley, and chill. Serve with warm pita bread and fresh vegetables.

Mellow Hommus for Versatility

This basic hommus tastes great plain, but it can also be used as the base for any hommus you'd like to make. Other ingredients can include minced, roasted red peppers; minced sweet green peppers; a combination of minced red and green peppers; a combination of minced green peppers and scallions; scallions alone; ¼ cup fresh minced parsley and scallions; a combination of minced jalapeño and red peppers; or jalapeño alone.

    1 can chickpeas, washed and drained (save the liquid)
    3 cloves garlic, minced
    3 tablespoons lemon juice
    ¼ cup water
    3 teaspoons tahini
    ½ teaspoon paprika
    2 tablespoons olive oil

Preparation. Combine all ingredients in food processor or chopper and process until smooth. For a creamier consistency, add additional olive oil, or liquid from the chickpeas. Garnish with fresh parsley sprigs.

CHAPTER 10

Sumptuous Green Salads and Fresh Salad Dressings

Greens and herbal energy are a powerful combination for flavor, vitality, fiber, and health. You can toss in fresh chive flowers for a dash of purple, yellow dandelion flowers for a touch of sunshine, or chrysanthemum flowers, which are a "long life" blessing.

Fresh Herbal Croutons

Make your own herbal croutons from fresh bread. Toast two slices of fresh bread to crispy brown. Use a long knife to cut the toast into chunks or cubes. You can also use quick raps with a pestle to break the toast into small chunks or crumbs to sprinkle over a salad. Think of the options that fresh bread will give you for more vivid croutons: pumpernickel croutons, sourdough croutons, sunflower and flax croutons, eight-grain croutons, rye croutons, and oat bran croutons. What about banana bread croutons, pumpkin bread croutons, and zucchini bread croutons? A world of pleasure can perk up your everyday salads.

TO HERBALIZE CROUTONS, shake the croutons in a paper bag with your favorite herbs.

BUTTERY HERBAL CROUTONS. Lightly sauté toasted croutons in a teaspoon of butter with your favorite herbs.

Ready-to-Eat Salads

I like salads that are ready to eat, so I chop greens into bite-size pieces. That way, each bite with dressing has a more harmonious blend.

Honey Spread for Sweetening

A nice touch for smooth sweetening with honey is to use a honey spread, which has a smoother consistency and often has a lighter color than standard honey and makes sweetening with honey a dream. The one I use comes from Rutland, Massachusetts: George Gershman's crystallized clover honey spread, which also contains royal jelly, one of the greatest healers known. Clover honey is available at natural health food stores (or write P.O. Box 687, Rutland, MA, 01543). There are many versions of honey spreads in natural grocery stores, which give you a variety of flavors and an even consistency when you sweeten with honey. Explore the possibilities, and support your local honey makers—they care about the quality of honey for your health.

Fresh Salad Dressings

The subtle flavor of a fresh salad dressing is unbeatable, and you can significantly reduce your sugar intake by making a few fresh salad dressings to keep on hand. Fresh dressings enrich the flavor and blend of the herbs and spices and give you pure energy you can feel at the first taste.

For ease and convenience, make oily fresh salad dressings in small glass jars, cover, mildly shake to blend, and chill. Serve the dressing separately in a cruet, and save the remaining dressing in the jar. Blend creamy dressings in a bowl, and store them in jars or plastic containers to have on hand for salads. When you keep your greens and dressings separate, your greens stay crisper and keep better when you refrigerate greens for the next day. Your salad dressings are versatile, too. They can be used as dips for vegetables or as toppings for pasta and rice, and an oily dressing can be used as a fresh marinade or to baste chicken, pork, lamb, and fish.

✌ *Green Goddess Dressing*

The green goddess, parsley, meets a few friends for a fabulous get-together with a rich taste and powerful health benefits, including antioxidants. This also makes a great topping or dip.

½ cup chopped fresh parsley

1½ tablespoons fresh tarragon leaves (¾ teaspoon dried)

3 tablespoons chopped fresh chives (1½ tablespoons dried)

1 clove garlic, crushed

1 or 2 anchovies

½ cup mayonnaise

½ cup sour cream

1 tablespoon tarragon vinegar

2 tablespoons water

Preparation. Combine all ingredients in a blender, and blend until smooth. Makes 1 cup. Keeps for one to two weeks. Stir the blend each time you use it.

✌ *Fresh Thousand Island Dressing*

This creamy blend has a subtle harmony of vegetables and spices, and it includes protein! It also makes a great topping or dip. Makes 1 cup.

½ cup yogurt
½ cup sour cream
3 teaspoons minced green pepper
8 green olives with pimientos
2 teaspoons diced green chiles (canned)
1 teaspoon paprika
½ teaspoon chile powder
¼ teaspoon honey (or honey spread)
Dash of cinnamon
1 hard-boiled egg
Dash of salt to taste

Preparation. Combine yogurt and sour cream. Mince pepper, green olives, and green chiles in a chopper, and add to yogurt blend. Add paprika, chile powder, honey, and cinnamon. Mince egg in the chopper separately and fold into blend. Chill. The blend peaks after it is chilled. If you would like more zest, add more paprika or a dash of salt.

❧ *Roasted Red Pepper Vinaigrette*

¼ cup Roasted Red Pepper Puree (see recipe in chapter 8)
¼ cup red wine vinegar or red raspberry vinegar
⅛ cup olive oil
⅛ cup fresh orange juice (clementines are superb)

Preparation. Combine ingredients in a jar. Shake to blend, and chill.

❧ *Mediterranean Medley Vinaigrette*

Red raspberry vinegar and orange mingle with Mediterranean herbs to give you a lift of pleasure.

¼ cup olive oil
½ cup red raspberry vinegar
6 black olives, minced
2 teaspoons fresh chives, minced (or parsley)
½ teaspoon dried oregano
1 clove garlic, minced
1 teaspoon onion, minced
1 teaspoon dried thyme
Juice of 1 whole orange (or 2–3 clementines)
¼ teaspoon honey (or honey spread) to taste

Preparation. Combine olive oil and raspberry vinegar in a jar. In a chopper or blender, combine olives, chives, oregano, garlic, onion, and thyme. Add to blend. Add juice of orange and honey, and shake. If you like it tangy, leave out the honey.

❦ EZ Blue Cheese Dressing

¼ cup crumbled blue cheese
½ cup plain yogurt

Preparation. Combine and spin it in a chopper or whip to blend.

❦ Feta Cheese Dressing

Feta Cheese Dressing is great on any greens, and you can use it on vegetables, fish, or crackers, and as stuffing for chicken.

4 ounces cream cheese (or yogurt cheese)
4 ounces feta, crumbled
⅓ cup mayonnaise
1 clove garlic, minced
¼ teaspoon basil
¼ teaspoon oregano
⅛ teaspoon thyme

Preparation. Blend and chill.

❦ Creamy Orange Nectar Dressing

Low-fat yogurt and low-fat sour cream work splendidly for this dressing. It also makes a fabulous sauce on fruit.

½ cup plain yogurt (low-fat works well)
½ cup sour cream
½ teaspoon honey (or honey spread)
Juice of 1 orange

Preparation. Combine ingredients, blend, and chill.

🌿 *Cinnamon Nectar*

Oh so sweet and creamy, even with low-fat yogurt and sour cream. You can use this on anything from greens to fruits, as a sweet sandwich spread, or as a topping on fish.

 ½ cup yogurt
 ½ cup sour cream
 ½ teaspoon honey (or honey spread)
 ½ teaspoon cinnamon

Preparation. Combine and spin it in a chopper or whip to blend.

🌿 *Sweet Honey-Mustard Mayonnaise*

You get the rich taste of mayonnaise in a mellow blend. You can add a green herb to this blend as well—such as chives, marjoram, tarragon, or savory. Also experiment with your favorite mustard blends.

 ¼ cup sour cream
 2 teaspoons mayonnaise
 ¼ teaspoon honey (or honey spread)
 ¼ teaspoon creamy mustard

Preparation. Combine and blend.

🌿 *Honey Yogurt Dressing*

This is an extremely versatile blend that makes a great salad dressing, topping, or dip for vegetables, fruit, chicken, or fish.

    ¼ cup sour cream
    ¼ cup yogurt
    ¼–½ teaspoon honey (or honey spread)

Preparation. Combine and blend.

Sumptuous Salads

🌿 *Pesto Surprise! Stuffed Tomato with Goat Cheese Broiled*

Make this exquisite treat for someone special—like yourself. It's a glorious appetizer for an elegant dinner with a light, white fish for the main meal. If you have a friend who loves pesto, serve it as a salad for lunch.

    1 small tomato
    ½ cup of pesto
    ¼–½ cup crumbled goat cheese (or slices)

Preparation. Slice top off of the tomato to remove dent, and level the rim of the tomato. Cut *V*s along the top rim of the tomato to let the pesto drip over the sides when it broils. Stuff tomato with pesto (see Pesto with Pine Nuts recipe in chapter 9). Surround the tomato with goat cheese in a small, round, low-rimmed oven-safe dish. Broil for 3–5 minutes.

🌿 *Pear Pecan Salad with Mediterranean Medley Dressing*

Pure decadence. The arrangement is part of the art.

  1 cup baby spinach
  Dash of coarsely ground pepper
  ¼ cup crumbled goat cheese
  ½ cup red onion, sliced in rings
  1 pear, sliced in quarters
  6 pecans dipped in honey, halved

Preparation. Arrange baby spinach carefully on plate and lightly pepper. Sprinkle goat cheese on spinach. Arrange onion rings around sides. Place pear slices in center. Dot half of the honeyed pecan slices on the pear slices, and dot the rest here and there. Drizzle with Mediterranean Medley Vinaigrette (recipe at the start of this chapter). You may find you have to fan yourself after the first taste. You can also use your favorite bottled dressing.

🌿 *Forest-Green Salad with Shrimp and Fresh Thousand Island Dressing*

Three great greens combine to give this tossed salad stunning health benefits. You want to dice the shrimp so it snuggles with the greens in every bite. You get valuable antioxidants in parsley and watercress.

  ½ cup parsley, minced
  ½ cup watercress leaves, minced
  4 cups fresh spinach
  1 dozen shrimp, diced

Preparation. Remove stems from spinach. (If shrimp is frozen, cook in boiling water with a pinch of sea salt for 3 minutes, until tender. Remove shells and tails.) Cut spinach and shrimp into bite-sized pieces. Combine shrimp, spinach, parsley, and watercress and chill. Drizzle with Fresh Thousand Island Dressing (recipe at the start of this chapter) or your favorite bottled dressing.

Festival Salad with Broiled Chicken

A burst of color and taste sensations. Looks and tastes fabulous. This is one large salad for dinner or two small salads. Top with your favorite dressing or Roasted Red Pepper Vinaigrette (recipe at the start of this chapter).

½ cup red romaine, small pieces
½ cup curly endive, small pieces
½ cup cucumbers, sliced thin
½ cup baby tomatoes
½ cup red onion, sliced in rings
½–1 cup cooked chicken slices
1 teaspoon chile powder
2 teaspoons butter
½ cup pineapple bits

Preparation. Alternate the red and green lettuce on plate. Arrange cucumber slices around the edge of the salad, with tomatoes, remaining cucumbers, and onions alternating in center area. Broiled chicken: Use leftover chicken or precooked chicken tenders or strips. Cut chicken in strips. Combine 1 teaspoon chile powder with 2 teaspoons butter and baste chicken pieces with blend. Broil for about 2 minutes to brown. Place chicken in center of salad with pineapple bits on top.

✎ Cucumber and Onion with EZ Blue Cheese Dressing

This simple salad is elegant and easy. Lots of cucumber, sliced paper-thin, layered with onion, sliced paper-thin, too.

    2 leaves of red romaine lettuce
    1 small cucumber, sliced paper-thin
    ½ medium onion, sliced paper-thin
    2 teaspoons lemon juice
    ½ teaspoon lemon pepper

Preparation. Place red romaine lettuce on plate. Alternate cucumber and onion, drizzle with lemon juice, and follow with lemon pepper. Use EZ Blue Cheese Dressing (recipe at the start of this chapter).

✎ Mandarin Sesame Tossed Salad and Orange Nectar Dressing

Greens and citrus blend with a crunchy sesame flavor and nuts, with a sweet orange dressing to top it off.

    4 cups baby spinach, cut into bite-sized pieces
    1 cup mushrooms, sliced thin
    Optional: ¼ cup water chestnuts, chopped
    ¼ cup unsalted cashews, chopped
    ½ cup (or 1 small can) baby mandarin orange segments
    ¼ cup toasted sesame seeds

Preparation. Combine spinach leaves and sliced mushrooms. Sprinkle chopped water chestnuts and cashews over top. Add orange segments whole. Toast sesame seeds in a warm, dry frying pan to light brown (1 minute). Sprinkle over salad and toss. Use Orange Nectar Dressing (recipe at the start of this chapter).

Greens and Tomatoes and Feta Cheese Dressing

1–2 cups of any plain greens, or a combination
2 sliced tomatoes

Use greens liberally with a hearty dollop of Feta Cheese Dressing nested in the center of the greens. Surround the dressing with lots of tomatoes for pleasure and healing power.

Avocado Salad and Honey Yogurt Dressing

1 leaf red lettuce
2 tomatoes, sliced thin
1 ripe avocado, sliced thin
¼ Bermuda onion, diced
1–2 cloves garlic, diced
Dash of cayenne
2 tablespoons lemon juice (or lime)

Preparation. Place lettuce on plate; alternate tomato and avocado slices on lettuce. Combine onion, garlic, and cayenne, and chop in a chopper. Sprinkle over salad. Drizzle with lemon juice, and nest a dollop of Honey Yogurt Dressing in the center. See Honey Yogurt Dressing (recipe at the start of this chapter).

Turkey Walnut Salad with Dill

A citrus lift adds zest to leftover turkey. Serve on a bed of baby spinach. Serves 2.

2 cups diced turkey
1 cup mayonnaise (or ½ cup plain yogurt with ½ cup
    mayonnaise)
¼ cup walnuts, chopped
2 teaspoons fresh dill, chopped (or 1 teaspoon dried)
Bed of baby spinach
Salt and pepper to taste
1 small can mandarin oranges, drained

Preparation. Blend all ingredients except oranges. Use oranges whole, fold in gently.

🌿 *Tangy Carrot Salad*

This salad is sweet and tangy and easy to make. It makes its own dressing. Parsley and garlic have antioxidant and anti-inflammatory benefits to guard your heart and health, and pepper is a great digestive aid. Serves 4.

Bed of Boston lettuce
2 cloves garlic
½ bunch fresh parsley, chopped
2 large carrots, chopped
2 tablespoons lemon juice
2 tablespoons orange juice
2 tablespoons olive oil
Salt to taste
¼ teaspoon pepper (or to taste)

Preparation. Arrange lettuce on plate. In a food processor or chopper, combine garlic and parsley and chop. Add carrots, lemon juice, orange juice, olive oil, salt, and pepper. Grind or pulse until carrots are well chopped but not pureed. Serve the salad on Boston lettuce.

CHAPTER 11

Sandwich Haven

You can use wraps, pitas, or sliced bread for these herb-rich sandwich recipes. Wraps come in a variety of flavors—tomato, spinach, jalapeño, and wheat, to name just a few. Have fun with the assorted varieties, which can lend a different flavor to your sandwiches for different days.

Deluxe Greek Pita

This is the way to lunch for energy—lots of vegetables and herbs in one sandwich.

> 1 teaspoon olive oil
> ½ cup cucumber, sliced fine
> ½ cup chopped tomatoes
> ¼–½ cup crumbled feta
> ½ cup chopped parsley
> ¼ cup red onion, minced (or ½ cup for extra zest)
> 1 clove garlic, minced
> ¼ teaspoon dried basil (or ½ teaspoon fresh)
> ¼ teaspoon dried oregano
> ⅛ teaspoon dried thyme

Preparation. Drizzle 1 teaspoon of olive oil inside pita. Set aside cucumbers, tomatoes, and feta. Combine other ingredients in a chopper or blender and mince. Blend the tomatoes and cucumbers in the mix by hand to avoid mushy texture. Fill the pita and top it with feta.

✌ Southwest Salsa Pita

Another great vegetable and herb combo. All-energy, low fat—with protein in the cheese.

    ¼ cup shredded cheddar
    ½ cup chopped tomatoes
    2 teaspoons lime juice
    ¼ cup red onion, minced
    1 clove garlic, minced
    ½ jalapeño pepper, minced
    ½ cup fresh cilantro leaves, chopped (or parsley)

Preparation. Put everything (except cheddar, tomatoes, and lime juice) in a food processor or chopper, and chop. Transfer to bowl. Drizzle with lime juice. Chop tomatoes by hand and blend in gently. Taste test. Want it hotter? Add the other half of the jalapeño. Fill a pita and top it with shredded cheddar.

✌ Beans and Beef Pita

A hearty blend that is so satisfying. Make two pitas or chill half of the blend. It also makes a great snack on its own.

    1 cup ground beef   1 teaspoon olive oil
    2 cloves garlic, diced   1 small can baked beans
    1 teaspoon   1 teaspoon coriander
       dried thyme   ½ teaspoon cumin

Preparation. Sauté beef, garlic, and thyme in olive oil. Heat 1 small can of baked beans (vegetarian or regular); add coriander and cumin to the beans. Combine beans and beef and blend. Fill a pita. Add shredded lettuce, if you like.

Feature

🌿 *Three-Herb Sandwich Bread*

Three great herbs—basil, dill, and oregano—make this bake-at-home bread something to savor. It toasts like a dream—aromatic and crunchy.

This bread is made peasant style: no fuss, and lots of kneading—6 minutes—but after that, you set it aside, and the dough does the work on its own. You let it rise twice, then shape it into a ball that's ready to bake. It's minimal work for maximum pleasure. It's low in salt and sugar, but you'd never guess it from the rich taste. By the way, kneading dough is a great stress release if you put on some music and let yourself get into it.

½ cup diced onion	1 teaspoon salt
3 tablespoons butter	1 tablespoon sugar
1 cup and 2 tablespoons milk	3 cups all-purpose flour (plus ½ cup on the side)
½ teaspoon basil	¼ ounce (1 package) dry yeast (active)
½ teaspoon dill	
½ teaspoon oregano	

Preparation. Heat oven to 375 degrees. Sauté onion in butter until the onion is transparent. Let it cool thoroughly (8–10 minutes). Warm the milk on the stove, just to boiling, then turn off heat. In a mixing bowl, combine cooled onion, milk, and remaining ingredients and blend vigorously until smooth. Add just enough extra flour to form a soft dough. Flour a board and knead the dough thoroughly to make it smooth and elastic. (Stay with it for about 6 minutes.) Place the dough in a greased bowl, and turn it a few times to be sure that all sides are greased. Cover the bowl, set it in a warm place, and wander off for 45 minutes. Return—the dough will have doubled in size. Pound the dough down, shape it into a ball, and place it on a greased baking sheet. Cover it and wander off for 45 minutes. Return—the dough will have doubled in size again. Now it's ready to bake.

Bake the ball of bread for 25 to 30 minutes, or until browned on top. Remove it from the oven, brush with melted butter, and let it cool. This bread is a special treat for any sandwich, toasted or plain.

Three-Herb Bread Versatility: You can change the three herbs to your favorites to achieve a different taste each time you make the bread.

Deluxe Chicken Salad

Serve on toast with lettuce, tomato, and mayonnaise. Or fill a pita with ½ cup chopped cilantro, parsley, or shredded lettuce, spoon the chicken salad in, and top with sliced tomatoes. This chicken salad also makes a fine salad on its own on any bed of lettuce.

½ cup chopped onion
2 cloves garlic, chopped
2 teaspoons fresh parsley, chopped
2 cups diced chicken
1 teaspoon thyme
1 teaspoon chile powder
2 teaspoons mayonnaise to blend
Salt and pepper to taste

Preparation. Combine onion, garlic, and parsley in a bowl. Add chicken, thyme, chile powder, and mayonnaise, and blend. Salt and pepper to taste.

🌿 *Light and Delicate Egg Salad Sandwich*

A refreshing taste with a hint of green pepper. Try it in a jalapeño wrap or serve on toast with shredded lettuce and sliced tomatoes, with a mustard spread for zest. This recipe gives you a hearty amount, so you can chill it for protein snacks or serve it as a salad on a bed of greens.

 6 eggs
 3 tablespoons mayonnaise
 1 tablespoon green pepper, minced
 1 tablespoon onion, minced
 1 clove garlic, diced (or ½ teaspoon dried)
 Salt and pepper to taste

Preparation. Add a dash of white vinegar to the water for your hard-boiled eggs to keep the shells from cracking. Simmer your hard-boiled eggs for approximately 5 minutes, instead of boiling them, for a fresher taste. Chop eggs and whites fine, combine ingredients, and blend.

🌿 *The Portabella Burger*

A veggie burger that's easy to make, with a balsamic taste. Makes 2 burgers or 1 whopper.

 1 teaspoon butter
 1 teaspoon olive oil
 2 cloves garlic, diced
 1 large portabella mushroom, sliced in half

Preparation. Combine butter and olive oil and sauté garlic and both sides of portabella until tender but crisp. A minute before you remove the slices from the heat, hit each slice with ¼ teaspoon balsamic vinegar to peak the flavor. Serve on toast with sliced tomatoes, and try this spread for a hint of sweetness:

> Honey Mayo Spread
> 2 tablespoons mayonnaise
> ¼ teaspoon honey

Combine ingredients and blend. You can also add a dash of quality mustard to the Honey Mayo Spread for zest.

✿ Turkey Burger

This turkey burger is spiced up to taste like beef. Lots of flavor with half the fat of lean hamburger meat. This recipe gives you burgers to freeze. They defrost quicker than beef.

1 small red onion, chopped	1 teaspoon lemon pepper
¼ cup fresh parsley, chopped	½ teaspoon olive oil
2 cloves garlic, minced	2–4 teaspoons tomato paste
2 teaspoons chile powder	Dash of salt
1 teaspoon allspice	1 pound ground turkey

Preparation. Combine all ingredients except turkey meat in chopper and mince. Blend the mix from the chopper into the meat with your hands. Form into patties and freeze the extra burgers. They defrost in a flash for quick lunches. Serve on toast with sliced tomatoes and any green *Magic Teaspoon* creamy puree blend (see chapter 8). I like my burger with a dollop of Garlic Whammo as a spread, or try Roasted Red Pepper Puree in cream cheese as a spread.

✣ Chile Burger

Lots of zest without too much heat. If you want to make extra burgers to freeze, use 1 pound of meat and adjust the ingredients this way: 2 times each herb, but not more than ¼ cup red onion. Use the chile powder to garnish the outside of each patty before freezing. You can also crumble a cooked burger and fill a pita, with shredded lettuce and sliced tomatoes.

1 patty lean ground beef
2 garlic cloves, crushed
2 teaspoons red onion, chopped
1 teaspoon thyme
½ teaspoon lemon pepper
Dash of salt
1 teaspoon chile powder
1 teaspoon butter

Preparation. Combine all ingredients except chile powder. Form patty. Sprinkle ½ teaspoon chile powder on each side. Fry in 1 teaspoon butter. If you broil or grill, baste each side with a dash of butter first, and sprinkle chile powder on top. Serve on toast or bun with sliced tomatoes and your favorite spread or cheese.

✣ Coriander Burger with Swiss

An exotic taste that's deep and pleasing. You can use this for a pita by crumbling the burger and topping with chopped tomatoes and the Swiss cheese cut in strips.

1 patty lean ground beef
2 teaspoons red onion, chopped
2 cloves garlic, mashed
1 teaspoon coriander
½ teaspoon cumin
1 teaspoon thyme
Dash of salt and pepper
1 teaspoon butter
1 slice Swiss cheese

Preparation. Combine all ingredients except cheese and form a patty. Fry in 1 teaspoon butter, or broil or grill. Flip and top with cheese. Serve on toasted pumpernickel or bun with a bevy of sliced tomatoes.

Burger Tricks

- Fresh herbs work best in burgers when they are chopped very fine.

- *Cheese Surprise*. After blending herbs and spices in the beef, tuck a teaspoon of white cheese—feta, mozzarella, goat, or Brie—into the center of the patty before flattening. Fry, grill, or broil.

- *Puree Surprise*. Tuck 1 teaspoon of Dill Deliverance, Garlic Whammo, or Basil Bliss (see chapter 8) in the center of the meat before flattening.

- *Herb It Up*. Use lots of herbs in small amounts—thyme, sage, basil, rosemary, tarragon, marjoram, oregano—in any combination that pleases you.

- When grilling, set grill to highest heat, or heat coals to maximum heat before putting patties on. Watch closely so you don't overcook.

- Use ¼ cup fresh chopped cilantro and a squeeze of lime in your burger for south-of-the-border tang.

Light and Fancy Sandwich Fare

✇ *Creamy Walnut, Chives, and Watercress*

A luxurious blend that you can serve open-faced on toast or as a wrap. The key is to mince all of the ingredients to achieve a smooth blend.

    1 hard-boiled egg, minced
    ¼ cup walnuts, minced
    4 teaspoons watercress, minced
    2 teaspoons fresh chives, minced
    Salt and pepper to taste
    3 teaspoons mayonnaise

Preparation. Mix together egg, walnuts, watercress, chives, and a dash of salt and pepper with a quick spin in a food processor or blender. Fold into mayonnaise.

✇ *Cucumbers on Toast with Cinnamon Nectar Spread*

Toast your favorite bread and get ready for a sweet surprise! Serve open-faced.

    ½ small cucumber, sliced very thin, lightly salted

Cinnamon Nectar Spread
4 teaspoons yogurt
4 teaspoons sour cream
Dash of honey (or honey spread)
Dash of cinnamon

Preparation. Layer cucumbers on toast slices. Comine nectar ingredients, spoon nectar on top of cucumbers, and serve open-faced.

Cream Cheese, Chives, and Olives

There's extra tang in this classic. Serve open-faced.

¼ cup cream cheese (or yogurt cheese)
4 teaspoons snipped fresh chives (or two teaspoons dried, crushed)
¼ cup black or green olives with pimientos, sliced thin

Preparation. Combine cream cheese and chives. Spread the blend on pumpernickel and top with sliced olives.

Yellow Pepper and Basil on English Muffin

Indulge in luxury! Lots of pepper crowned with the king of the herbs, fresh basil leaves. Serve open-faced.

1 English muffin
2 teaspoons mayonnaise
8 thin slices fresh yellow peppers (small, sweet yellow peppers—superb)
2 large leaves fresh basil, or 4–6 small

Preparation. Toast English muffin and spread with mayonnaise. Press fresh pepper slices into the mayonnaise. Top with fresh basil leaves.

🌿 *Brie and Rosemary Grilled*

Use soft Brie beneath the hard covering for this recipe, and serve on pumpernickel bread.

    ¼ cup Brie
    1 teaspoon fresh rosemary leaves
    Optional: 1 teaspoon quality mustard spread on pumpernickel

Preparation. Spread soft Brie on bread slices. Press fresh chopped rosemary leaves into Brie. Broil for 1 to 2 minutes to lightly brown cheese. Serve open-faced.

🌿 *Herbed Monterey Jack*

Any great white bread—Italian, sourdough, or French—will work with this combination, but the Three-Herb Sandwich Bread (see recipe earlier in this chapter) tops the list.

    2 teaspoons chopped fresh parsley
    1 teaspoon fresh tarragon leaves (or ½ teaspoon dried)
    Dash of olive oil
    4 thin slices of tomatoes
    4 thin slices Monterey Jack (bar cheese)
    1 teaspoon butter, melted

Preparation. Mince parsley and tarragon and blend together in a dash of olive oil. Spread the herb blend on each slice of bread. Top with sliced tomatoes and cheese. Close sandwich. Brush the outsides with butter, and brown in frying pan. You can also broil this open-faced.

CHAPTER 12

Veggie Versatility

Never Again the Same Taste in Vegetables

When you enhance the flavor of your daily vegetables with vivid herbs and spices, vegetables are never boring, never bland, and the versatility they can bring to your menu is astounding. You may find that you crave vegetables more often and eat a wider variety simply because they taste so splendid with herbs and spices.

This adventure in healing pleasure with vegetables gives you two recipes for each vegetable, using a different herb or spice for each recipe, to show you how your old favorites can take on a different personality by using different herbs and spices.

Unlike other recipes where the ingredients are set, plain vegetables give you lots of room to experiment with herbs and spices that you might want to use for specific health problems that you'd like to improve. "The All-Naturals Guide" (chapter 4) will show you at a glance which herbs and spices are antacids, anti-inflammatories, antioxidants, digestive aids, depression fighters, blood builders, and more. You can use the guide to select herbs and spices that meet your health needs. For instance, you might struggle with nagging digestive distress, and "The All-Naturals Guide" will target herbs like allspice, fennel, and ginger as natural support to fight digestive disorders. If you struggle with depression and tension, you can target herbs like basil, chives, and dill, which strengthen your nervous system and help to ease stress, tension, and depression. It's a win–win combination in your everyday menu.

Look for Veggie Crisps at the end of this chapter. They taste like gourmet blends, but they take only one minute to prepare, and they cook themselves in the oven. It can't get easier than this to enhance your health with quick-cook recipes for vegetables, even the time-consuming ones like eggplant, zucchini, and squash.

An easy way to find the antioxidants in vegetables, herbs, and spices is to say "ACE": vitamins A, C, and E are the antioxidants. They're the latest newsmakers because they help to fight diseases of aging and cancer.

Artichokes

A low-sodium, low-calorie vegetable, artichokes are an excellent source of fiber—approximately 12 percent of your daily requirement—for intestinal health and a good source of protein. They provide essential minerals, including potassium, calcium, iron, and magnesium, and contain two antioxidants, vitamins A and C, along with B-complex for a healthy nervous system. Research indicates that artichokes also contain silymarin, a compound that protects the liver from damage by free radicals and toxins, and it can renew liver cells. Artichokes have no fat and no cholesterol. Jerusalem artichokes provide a natural source of insulin to help fight diabetes.

❧ *Artichoke Hearts with Honey-Mustard Dip*

Use artichoke hearts in a can or jar. Drain off liquid. For your dip, combine ¼ cup yogurt, 1 teaspoon mayonnaise, ½ teaspoon honey (or honey spread), ½ teaspoon quality creamy mustard, a dash of lemon pepper, and blend.

❧ *Artichoke Hearts with Honey Orange Sauce*

Use artichoke hearts in can or jar. Drain off liquid. Combine ¼ cup yogurt, ¼ cup sour cream, ¼ teaspoon honey (or honey spread), and the juice of 1 orange for a sweet, creamy sauce.

Asparagus

This is an ACE vegetable, with all three antioxidants: vitamins A, C, and E. It also contains B-complex, calcium, potassium, phosphorus, sulfur for skin health, iron for blood building, iodine for the thyroid, silicon, and rutin, a bioflavonoid that helps to fight cancer. Asparagus spears are excellent for your kidneys, bladder, and heart.

❧ *Spears Rosemary*

Lightly cook spears in a small amount of water until tender. Sprinkle with lemon pepper for zest. Separately sauté 2 teaspoons of butter and 1 teaspoon fresh rosemary (or ½ teaspoon dried and crushed). Spoon the blend over your spears just before you take them off the heat.

🌿 *Spears and Toasted Poppy Seeds*

Lightly cook spears in a small amount of water until tender. Separately sauté 1 teaspoon poppy seeds in 2 teaspoons butter in a frying pan to burst their flavor (1–2 minutes). Spoon the blend over your spears for a rich, nutty flavor.

Beets

The maroon beetroot is high in potassium (343 mg in 1 cup) and calcium, and low in sodium. It's also a red blood builder with iron. It's a natural alkalizer and body cleanser with vitamins A, B-complex, and C, magnesium, and phosphorus. Fresh beets are fabulous! Precook a batch of whole fresh beets until tender (½ hour). Remove skin and dice. Chill the extra for later.

🌿 *Pickled Beet Salad—Zesty*

Sauté ¼ cup diced red onion in 2 teaspoons olive oil with 1 bay leaf, until onion is transparent. Add to 1 cup diced beets, and top with ¼ cup red wine vinegar (or red raspberry vinegar). Chill in a jar. Remove bay leaf before serving.

🌿 *Beets and Allspice*

A combination with a deep, rich flavor. In small saucepan, heat 4 teaspoons butter and 2 teaspoons allspice, stirring to blend. Add 1 cup diced beets, and blend thoroughly. Serve hot or chilled.

Broccoli

A low-fat vegetable that is high in the antioxidant vitamin A, broccoli helps to fight cancer. It's a good source of calcium (132 mg in 1 cup), and protein (4.6 grams), and it contains potassium, iron, magnesium, phosphorus, and vitamin C.

✿ *Broccoli, Baby Bella, and Garlic*

Steam 1 cup broccoli florets in 1 cup water until tender. In 2 teaspoons butter, sauté ½ cup sliced baby bella mushrooms, 1 clove fresh chopped garlic, and 1 teaspoon lemon pepper, stirring to blend. Pour mushrooms and sauce over warm broccoli.

See Veggie Crisps at the end of this chapter for your second broccoli recipe.

Brussels Sprouts

These sprouts give you power (5.5 grams of protein in one cup). They're also high in vitamin A (676 IU), vitamin C (113 mg), potassium (355mg), and phosphorus (94 mg). They also contain magnesium, iron, niacin, riboflavin, calcium, and the fiber cellulose—to increase your food transit time and flush toxins.

✿ *Beyond Brussels Sprouts*

Cook 1 cup of sprouts in a small amount of salted water until tender but crisp, and drain. Combine ¼ cup sour cream, ¼ cup yogurt, ½ teaspoon honey (or honey spread), and ½ teaspoon cinnamon. Spoon cold sauce over warm sprouts.

See Veggie Crisps at the end of this chapter for your second brussels sprouts recipe.

Cabbage

A valued cure-all since 400 BC, cabbage is anti-inflammatory, antibacterial, and antirheumatic, and it stimulates the production of new cells. For colitis, cabbage leaves were boiled to make a potent juice and taken as a liquid. It contains the fiber pectin, which helps to prevent blood sugar swings and helps to lower cholesterol. It also has potassium (277 mg), vitamin A (221 IU), vitamin C, B-complex, vitamin K, vitamin U (which fights ulcers), calcium, iodine, sulfur, iron, and protein. This combination helps to fight diseases, including cancer.

Purple Cabbage and Thyme

Remove core from cabbage, cut the cabbage into wedges, cook in water, covered, until tender, and drain. Combine 2 tablespoons olive oil, 1 teaspoon dried, crushed thyme, and ¼ teaspoon lemon pepper, and simmer, stirring to blend. Pour over 1 cup of cabbage. Store remaining cabbage for fabulous cold snacks.

Chilled Purple Cabbage and Marjoram

Combine ¼ cup of red raspberry vinegar with 1 teaspoon dried, crushed marjoram (or 2 teaspoons fresh). Pour over purple cabbage. You can use a variety of your favorite salad dressings and add one herb to freshen the dressing, varying the flavor every time you snack on chilled purple cabbage.

Carrots

The sweet orange roots are powerful health treats with one of the ACE antioxidants in high amounts—vitamin A—15,750 IU in one cup! They help to fight diseases of aging and cancer. Carrots also contain protein, calcium, iron, phosphorus, potassium, B-complex, vitamin C, iodine, and pectin to balance sugar swings and lower cholesterol.

✌ *Carrots and Nutmeg Blend*

These carrots taste like candy! Sauté 1 cup cooked, thin-sliced carrots in 2 teaspoons butter with ¾ teaspoon allspice and ¼ teaspoon nutmeg. Let them simmer for a few minutes to peak the exotic flavor.

✌ *Carrots and Dill*

Slice baby carrots in half. Combine 2 teaspoons butter and 1 teaspoon dried dill (or 2 teaspoons fresh, minced), add carrots, and let them simmer for a few minutes to mellow the flavor.

Cauliflower

Mark Twain called cauliflower a cabbage with a college education, because he thought it looked like a brain. The fancy white florets help to stabilize blood sugar and lower cholesterol with pectin. They also contain two of the ACE antioxidants, vitamin A (very high content) and vitamin C, which fight many major diseases, including cancer. Cauliflower has calcium for strong bones, iron for blood building, phosphorus, niacin, potassium, and vitamin B_1.

See Veggie Crisps at the end of this chapter for two cauliflower recipes that cook in a flash.

Corn

One cup of corn will give you 4.2 grams of protein, a boost of antioxidant power with vitamin A (540 IU), and potassium (194 mg). Corn also brings you phosphorus, magnesium, calcium, biotin, niacin, and iron for blood building. Keep in mind that it's higher in sodium than other vegetables, and that calls for some salt savvy.

Rev-It-Up Summer Corn on the Cob

Instead of salt, use butter and a sprinkling of Rev It Up: Combine 4 teaspoons dried parsley, 4 teaspoons dried dill, 2 teaspoons dried mustard powder, 1 teaspoon dried garlic powder, and 1 teaspoon cayenne pepper.

Winter Corn and Chives

Briefly heat frozen corn in water to defrost to tender, but crisp. Sauté 2 teaspoons butter and 2 teaspoons crushed dried chives for a summery flavor in winter.

Eggplant

This purple beauty is low in sodium, with calcium, iron, magnesium, phosphorus, potassium, and the antioxidant vitamin C, which fights diseases of aging and helps to prevent infections, including colds and flu.

See Veggie Crisps at the end of this chapter for two gourmet eggplant recipes that cook in a flash.

Green Beans

Green beans are an excellent source for two disease-fighting antioxidants, with high vitamin A (675 IU in one cup) and vitamin C. They also contain calcium, iron, phosphorus, potassium, magnesium, choline, vitamins B_1 and B_2, and two great fibers, cellulose and pectin, to keep you lean by increasing your food transit time while they stabilize your blood sugar and help to lower your cholesterol.

ℬ *Green Beans Italian*

Simmer 1 cup Italian (or your favorite) green beans in ½ cup water until tender, and drain. Combine 2 teaspoons olive oil, ¼ cup chopped red onion, and 2 teaspoons fresh lemon juice in a skillet. Add warm green beans and sauté to blend thoroughly (about 5 minutes).

ℬ *Sweet and Sour Green Beans*

Steam 1 cup of your favorite green beans until tender, and drain. Combine ¼ cup sour cream, ¼ cup yogurt, ½ teaspoon honey (or honey spread), and ¼ teaspoon cinnamon. Spoon the cold sauce over the warm beans.

Kale

Forest-green kale is low in fat, calories, and sodium and rich in antioxidant power with 7,400 IU of vitamin A in one cup, for cancer fighting and disease resistance. Kale also gives you 134 mg calcium, 221 mg potassium, and 68 mg of vitamin C, along with 3 grams of protein and a dash of niacin.

✇ *Kale with Onions, Almonds, and Allspice*

Cook and drain 1 box frozen kale. Drizzle with lemon juice. Combine kale with ½ cup chopped onions, 2 cloves garlic, chopped, ¼ cup chopped almonds, 2 teaspoons allspice, and ¼ teaspoon lemon pepper. Simmer until onions are transparent. If you want it sweet, add ¼–½ teaspoon honey.

✇ *Creamed Kale with Mustard Sauce*

Cook and drain 1 box frozen kale. Drizzle with lemon juice and salt. Cream sauce: Combine equal parts sour cream and yogurt (¼ cup each), 2 teaspoons creamy honey mustard, and a dash of lemon pepper. Add to warm kale and blend. To make your own honey mustard spread, combine ½ teaspoon honey (or honey spread) with 1 teaspoon of creamy mustard.

Mushrooms

Commonly used as a vegetable, this world-famous fungus is "meat" in vegetarian menus. They are 90 percent water, with iron, magnesium, potassium, niacin, and vitamin C, and they're higher in sodium than most vegetables.

✇ *Mushroom Caps with Onion, Fennel, and Thyme*

Combine ½ cup (or 1 small can) mushroom caps and ¼ cup chopped onions, and sauté in 2 teaspoons olive oil, with ½ teaspoon thyme and 1 teaspoon fennel.

See Veggie Crisps at the end of this chapter for gourmet mushroom caps that cook in a flash.

Onion

The bulb of this 6,000-year-old treasured herb was a staple in the diet of the pyramid builders for stamina and health. It's a four-star healer—antiseptic to fight infections, antibacterial, a tonic for the nerves, a soother for pain and trauma, and a rich source of the bioflavonoid quercetin, a cancer fighter. Onions also increase circulation, help to lower cholesterol, help to prevent clots, help to reduce high blood pressure, cleanse toxins from your system, and ease digestive difficulties. They also increase metabolic heat to burn fats. They're rich in vitamins A, B-complex, and C, high in sulfur (the health protector), and antirheumatic.

See Veggie Crisps at the end of this chapter for two gourmet onion recipes that cook in a flash.

Peppers

Sweet peppers are a good source of potassium, and they also contain magnesium, phosphorus, vitamins A and C—two major antioxidants to fight premature aging and cancer—niacin, and traces of vitamins B_1 and B_2.

See Veggie Crisps for Mexical Pepper Crisps and Red Pepper Two-Spice Crisps at the end of this chapter.

Spinach

An ancient herb from Persia, spinach is good for vision, the heart, and blood building, and an excellent vegetable for digestive strength. It's a rich source of iron, with chlorophyll to oxygenate cells, calcium to prevent intestinal polyps, the antioxidant vitamins A and C, as well as folic acid, phosphorus, potassium, and vitamin K.

✌ Dilled Spinach

Cook and drain 1 box frozen spinach. Sauté 2 tablespoons butter, 2 teaspoons dried dill, and a dash of lemon pepper. Mix in spinach. It tastes like instant pesto. Garlic lovers can add 1–2 cloves of fresh minced garlic to the sauté for extra pleasure and healing power.

✌ Crunchy Spinach with Toasted Poppy Seeds

Cook and drain 1 box frozen spinach. Drizzle with 1 teaspoon lemon juice and 2 teaspoons butter. Toast 2 teaspoons of poppy seeds in 2 teaspoons butter in a skillet. Pour over spinach.

Summer Squash

Squash is low in sodium and a good source of the antioxidant vitamin A. It also contains magnesium, phosphorus, potassium, niacin, and a second antioxidant in vitamin C, which fights colds, flu, and infections.

✌ Fried Squash and Garlic

Dredge in flour 1 cup of fresh summer squash cut in slender rounds. Fry in 2 teaspoons olive oil and 2 cloves garlic, chopped (or 1 teaspoon dried).

See Veggie Crisps at the end of this chapter for your second squash recipe that cooks in a flash.

Tomato

This red fruit that we use as a vegetable is a cancer fighter and anti-aging vegetable, rich in the antioxidant vitamin A (2,100 units) and the carotenoid lycopene, shown to reduce the risk of cancer of the prostate in a Harvard study on men. It's a good source of iron, and it contains phosphorus, potassium, niacin, and lots of water.

❧ Baked Tomatoes with Oregano

A lush tomato treat! Slice 3–4 tomatoes and place on a cookie sheet. Blend 4 teaspoons olive oil and 2 teaspoons dried oregano. Bake at 350 degrees for about 5 minutes. This is luxurious without cheese!

❧ Baked Tomatoes with Basil and Parmesan.

Slice 3–4 tomatoes and place on a cookie sheet. Combine 1 teaspoon dried basil with 2 teaspoons olive oil. Drizzle over tomatoes. Top with fresh grated Parmesan. Bake at 350 degrees for about 5 minutes.

Turnips

This sienna-colored root is a natural antacid. High in the antixodant vitamin A to fight disease, it also contains calcium, phosphorus, iron, sulfur, chlorophyll, and the antioxidant vitamin C. Turnips help to reduce high blood pressure.

❧ Buttery Turnips and Sage

Simmer 1 cup frozen turnip chunks in water until tender, and drain. Heat 2 teaspoons butter and blend in 1 teaspoon dried sage (or 2 teaspoons fresh) and a dash of lemon pepper. Pour over turnips. Delectable!

✒ *Buttery Turnips and Allspice*

Simmer 1 cup frozen turnip chunks in water until tender, and drain. Heat 2 teaspoons butter and blend in 2 teaspoons allspice. Pour over turnips.

Zucchini

This garden favorite is a zinger for fighting disease, loaded with the antioxidant vitamin A (7,000 IU), also calcium, iron, magnesium, phosphorus, potassium, and the antioxidant vitamin C.

See Veggie Crisps at the end of this chapter for gourmet zucchini that you can cook in a flash.

Feature: Veggie Crisps

Sizzle your way to pleasure with gourmet blends of vegetables, herbs, and spices that take one minute to prepare and cook themselves in the oven on high heat. Exciting and versatile vegetable blends can enhance your menu every day.

I prepared trays of veggie crisps, using different herbs or spices on one vegetable at a time, and used my taste testers to pick their favorites. On each vegetable listed below, everyone picked the same combination I preferred, so I'm confident that you'll like the choices, too. Everyone will find their own favorite crisps, but these were terrific!

Veggie crisps make excellent snacks, side dishes, and toppings for rice, pasta, fish, chicken, or beef. The versatility is phenomenal.

Simply by changing the herb or spice you choose to create your veggie crisps, you can vary the flavor of any vegetable each time you cook it, and choose the health benefits you'd like to receive.

How to Make Veggie Crisps

Preheat oven to 500 degrees. Cut your vegetable of choice into bite-sized chunks or wedges. In a wide-mouthed jar, combine 4 teaspoons of olive oil and 1 teaspoon of any dried herb or spice. The mixture will be thick. Add 1 cup of vegetable chunks to the jar. Cover the jar and shake until the vegetable chunks are fully coated. Bake on a cookie sheet or in a baking dish and let the vegetable sizzle for 8 to 10 minutes.

ONION CRISPS. The onions turn gold when they cook—use turmeric. Think of it! These onion crisps help to fight cancer. Golden onion crisps are also a luxurious topping for rice, pasta, or meat dishes. Slice an onion in quarters and peel the layers apart to form your crisps. They'll curl when they cook. To make healthy onion rings, cut the onion in half and peel the onion in rings to make the crisps. Add 1 teaspoon of turmeric to 4 teaspoons of olive oil in the jar.

EGGPLANT, MUSHROOM, OR ONION CRISPS. Use thyme or fennel to make the crisps flavor-rich. Add 1 teaspoon of thyme or fennel to 4 teaspoons of olive oil in the jar.

CAULIFLOWER OR ZUCCHINI CRISPS. Use allspice for a zesty flavor. Add 1 teaspoon of allspice to 4 teaspoons of olive oil in the jar.

SWEET PEPPERS (RED, ORANGE, GREEN), ONIONS, CAULIFLOWER, OR BROCCOLI make great Mexical Crisps with chile powder. Cut the vegetables in strips or chunks and combine red, green, and orange peppers in one jar, or peppers and onion in one jar, or cauliflower and broccoli. Add 1 teaspoon of chile powder to 4 teaspoons of olive oil in the jar.

ZUCCHINI, SWEET PEPPERS, ONIONS, OR BRUSSELS SPROUTS become Two-Spice Crisps with the team of nutmeg and allspice. Cut the vegetables in strips or chunks and add ¾ teaspoon allspice and ¼ teaspoon nutmeg to 4 teaspoons of olive oil in the jar.

SUMMER SQUASH OR MUSHROOMS develop a rich, exotic flavor with sage and lemon pepper. Add ¾ teaspoon sage and ¼ teaspoon lemon pepper to 4 teaspoons of olive oil in the jar.

ZUCCHINI, SUMMER SQUASH, MUSHROOMS, EGGPLANT, ONIONS, OR BROCCOLI get a garlic lift. Add 1 teaspoon dried garlic to 4 teaspoons of olive oil in the jar.

CHAPTER 13

Chilled Side Dishes and Snacking Sensations

You can add vital energy to your daily menu when you keep chilled vegetable and herb blends on hand for snacks and side dishes. They satisfy cravings and conquer hunger pangs with high-energy nutrition. These recipes take some of your old favorites to new heights of richness to inspire and delight you. They leave you feeling satisfied, refreshed, and pampered with pleasure.

✲ Sweet and Sassy Coleslaw

A dreamy and powerful health treat. Serves 4–6.

  ½ large cabbage (or 1 small), sliced fine or shredded
  2 carrots, sliced fine or shredded
  ¼ cup fresh parsley, chopped fine
  ¼ cup raisins (golden preferred, for color blend)
  2 cloves garlic, chopped
  4 teaspoons fresh dill (or 2 teaspoons dried dill)
  ¼ cup plain yogurt
  ¼ cup mayonnaise

Preparation. Make the coleslaw in bite-sized pieces, so every taste carries the sassy, sweet flavor. I withhold the yogurt and mayonnaise and blend smaller amounts into portions of the coleslaw just before I eat it, for a fresh blend. I also eat the coleslaw plain (with only a dash of mayonnaise) as a snack. When you chill coleslaw without the mayonnaise, it stays fresh for ten days.

Summer in a Bowl—Chilled Penette Salad

White, yellow, and light green are the tints in this pasta salad when it's blended. It's like summer in a bowl, and it's energizing like summer, vivid and adventurous, overflowing with nutrition, including protein. Makes 10 cups—and you'll probably need more!

1 medium box penette (baby pene, ziti, twirls, elbows, or bows)
2 tablespoons mayonnaise
2 tablespoons cider vinegar
1 teaspoon lemon pepper
2 teaspoons celery seeds
4 teaspoons milk
1 cup celery, chopped
1 cup fresh parsley, chopped
1 cup onion, chopped
4 hard-boiled eggs
½ cup green olives
2 teaspoons capers
Salt and pepper to taste

Preparation. Cook pasta al dente, drain, and return to pot. In a bowl, combine mayonnaise, vinegar, lemon pepper, celery seeds, and milk. Add to pasta and blend. Add celery, parsley, and onion to pasta and blend. Slice eggs and olives by hand; use whole capers—add to pasta and blend gently. Cover and chill for 1 hour. Taste test before you add salt or pepper.

✿ One Phenomenal Potato Salad

The taste of this potato salad is so exotic, you must experience it! Making the herbal blend is a delight in itself. From the first kiss of the olive oil and cider vinegar, you build a flavor and fragrance that intensifies with each new ingredient and peaks when you add the oregano. It's equally delicious hot or cold, with or without mayonnaise. Serves 6–8. Tastes even better the next day.

6 cups cooked red bliss potatoes, cut in chunks (or sliced)

Herbal Mix (Try it in this order to peak the fragrance)
½ cup olive oil
¼ cup cider vinegar
2 cloves garlic, mashed
½ cup black olives
¼ cup capers
¼ cup fresh chives (or 2 teaspoons dried)
1 cup Bermuda onion, chopped fine
2 teaspoons dried oregano (this is where the fragrance peaks)
1 teaspoon dried thyme leaves
2 teaspoons celery seeds
Salt and coarsely ground pepper to taste
Optional: ½ cup celery, chopped fine
⅓ cup mayonnaise*

*Note: Mayonnaise is added just before serving. Chilled potato salad stays fresher longer without the mayonnaise in the mix. Also, you might want to use it without mayonnaise as a side dish. For the whole dish, start with ⅓ cup mayonnaise, blend, and taste. You don't need a lot of mayonnaise with this beauty.

Preparation. Cook potato chunks in water, bring to a boil, reduce heat to medium, and simmer until soft for 10 to 15 minutes (pierce with a fork to test). Meanwhile, begin with the olive oil and cider vinegar in a bowl, and add the remaining ingredients except mayonnaise one by one. It goes quickly, and the fragrance keeps you invigorated. Add the bowl of ingredients to drained, hot potatoes, and blend lightly. Sample it hot! It's fabulous. Chill for a few hours, stirring occasionally. If you will be using the whole dish, just before serving, blend with ⅓ cup mayonnaise. If you will be using it over time, add mayonnaise to taste before each serving.

✒ *Delicate Deviled Eggs*

This recipe is a work of art when it's completed. Perfect for snacks, side dishes, or party platters. Makes 24 halves, and they'll go fast!

    12 eggs, hard-boiled
    2 heaping teaspoons mayonnaise
    3 teaspoons fresh onion, minced
    ½ teaspoon dry mustard
    ½ teaspoon garlic powder
    ½ teaspoon Tabasco sauce
    1 teaspoon Worcestershire sauce
    ½ teaspoon salt, or to taste
    6 olives with pimientos, halved
    Paprika

Preparation. Slice eggs in halves, remove yellows, and arrange whites on a tray. In bowl, crush yellows. Add all ingredients except olives and paprika, and blend. Taste test and add salt if you prefer. Spoon blend into egg whites level with eggs. Using a fork, create lengthwise ridges on the top of the egg blend. Garnish with ½ olive in the center, pimento facing up, and drizzle with paprika. Pretty as a picture.

🌿 Minty Parsley–Pea Salad, Chilled

Quick and delicious! A marvelous accompaniment for fish, particularly salmon. Great on its own, for an invigorating snack. Serves 4.

> 1 package frozen peas, thawed
> ½ cup fresh parsley, chopped
> 2 teaspoons fresh mint leaves (or 1 teaspoon dried)*
> ⅓ cup mayonnaise
> 3 teaspoons Dijon or other quality mustard
> 1–2 teaspoons horseradish sauce
> Salt and fresh ground pepper to taste

> *Note: You can use 2 teaspoons fresh chives (or 1 teaspoon dried) instead of mint, for variation.

Preparation. Mix ingredients and chill to blend flavors. Serve alone or on a bed of lettuce. Add more Dijon and horseradish sauce, if you like a lot of zest.

🌿 Old-World Tabbouleh

This Middle Eastern classic is pure perfection. It's a Lebanese family recipe that was handed down through generations. One taste wakes up your senses and fills you with energy, and it will keep you lean. Great for snacks, side dishes, as a topping for chicken or fish, and as a filling for sandwiches. You can also use this recipe as a base and add other vegetables and herbs for variations. For a classic Middle Eastern lunch, try Old-World Tabbouleh in a pita.

> ½ cup bulgur
> 2 cups fresh parsley, chopped fine
> Juice from 1 fresh lemon
>
> 2 teaspoons olive oil
> Salt and pepper to taste
> 1 tomato, diced fine

Preparation. Bulgur comes in an instant version or the extended version. Follow package directions to make. Combine parsley, lemon juice, olive oil, salt, and pepper in a chopper or blender to get a finely diced blend. Pour off any water that didn't absorb into the bulgur, add the bulgur to the chopper blend, and spin it briefly to blend it in. Add the finely diced tomato to the mix. Chill for 1 hour.

Quick Cold Pasta

Pasta salads have more vitality when you use lots of carrots as the base—and the beta-carotene helps to fight cancer.

    2 whole carrots, chopped fine
    ½ cup onion, chopped fine
    1 red pepper, chopped fine
    2 cloves garlic, chopped fine
    1 box ribbed ziti
    2 teaspoons dill, dried
    1 teaspoon celery salt
    ½ teaspoon salt
    4 hard-boiled eggs
    ¼ teaspoon pepper

Preparation. Toss together carrots, onion, red pepper, and garlic. Cook ziti al dente in 1 teaspoon dried dill, drain. Add 1 teaspoon dill, celery salt, salt, and pepper. Chop eggs by hand and blend gently into salad. Chill without dressing. This will let you use a different dressing each time you serve it. Creamy Parmesan and ranch are my favorite dressings on this pasta salad.

✿ Casual Cold Burrito Platter and Fresh Salsa Ingredients

This casual platter gives you a full meal with protein from the chicken and lots of nutrition from vegetables and herbs. Serve the vegetables in bite-sized pieces, in bowls, so family, friends, or guests can fashion their own festival of healthy food. It's a great way to turn leftover chicken into a fiesta.

Bowl of chicken pieces (strips)
6 tortilla wraps
Bowl of fresh lettuce, chopped
Bowl of fresh cilantro (or parsley), chopped
Bowl of 3 jalapeño chiles, minced
Bowl of tomatoes, chopped
Bowl of garlic cloves, chopped
Bowl of red onions, chopped
Bowl of cucumbers, diced
Bowl of olives (black, green, or both), sliced
Bowl of fresh shredded Parmesan
Bowl of lime quarters for lime juice

Preparation. Chicken: Baste chicken strips with a blend of butter and chile powder and broil on a tray until brown (2 minutes). You can also use the leftover chicken as is, without broiling, but give it a little zest with a drizzle of pepper, chile powder, or paprika.

CHAPTER 14

Hot Side Dishes

These rich vegetable and herb medleys can be your mainstay for heat-and-serve side dishes and snacks. Make them once, and store them for versatile uses.

Rata-tat-a-touille

This ratatouille has extra *ratatat*: high energy and low in calories with a fabulous flavor from the immunity booster basil. Make it as fresh as you can and store it for versatile uses: spoon it over rice, pasta, baked potatoes, chicken, or fish. Stuff it into a pita for a sandwich. Sprinkle it with Parmesan for a snack or side dish. Tastes great chilled, and reheats splendidly. Make it once and eat it all week.

2 whole eggplants,
    small to medium
4 yellow squash,
    small to medium
2 medium zucchini
1 onion, chopped
4 garlic cloves, chopped fine
4 teaspoons olive oil

6 fresh basil leaves, chopped
    fine (or 3 teaspoons dried)
10 plum tomatoes, chopped
    (or 1 large can peeled
    plum tomatoes with juice)
10 white mushrooms,
    medium to large, sliced
Salt and pepper to taste

Preparation. Slice eggplant, yellow squash, and zucchini into small chunks. In large saucepan, lightly brown onion and garlic in olive oil. Add eggplant chunks, basil, and plum tomatoes with juice. As vegetables begin to cook, add squash, zucchini, and sliced mushrooms. Salt and pepper to taste. Reduce heat to medium, and simmer until all vegetables are well cooked (15–20 minutes).

🌿 *Fancy French Green Bean Casserole*

Tastes as good as it looks, and it's easy to make. The cream sauce combines tarragon and mustard to create a flavor that sparkles. Serves 4–6.

> 1 teaspoon olive oil
> 1½ pounds frozen French green beans (1 package)
> ½ cup onion, diced
> 2 garlic cloves, diced
> 2 cups mushrooms, sliced
>
> *Herbal Cream Sauce*
> 2 tablespoons butter
> 3 tablespoons flour
> 1½ cups milk
> 2 teaspoons Dijon or other quality mustard
> 2 teaspoons dried tarragon
> Dash of salt and pepper to taste
> Optional: ½–¾ cup of breadcrumbs

Preparation. Preheat oven to 350 degrees. Grease a 2-quart casserole with olive oil and spread green beans over bottom of casserole dish. In food processor or chopper, mince onion and garlic. Add the onion–garlic mixture and the sliced mushrooms to the green beans. Drizzle with salt and pepper.

Herbal Cream Sauce: Over low heat, melt 2 tablespoons butter in saucepan. Gradually drizzle 3 tablespoons flour into butter, whisking to blend. Gradually add milk, whisking to blend. Bring to a light boil, and whisk until sauce thickens—2 minutes. Turn off heat. Blend in mustard and tarragon. Pour cream sauce over green beans and gently blend. Cover with bread crumbs. (See *Magic Teaspoon* Bread Crumbs for a zesty fresh recipe). Bake uncovered for 10 to 15 minutes, until bread crumbs are golden brown.

℀ *Magic Teaspoon Bread Crumbs*

2 slices bread
1 teaspoon butter
1 teaspoon tarragon
½ teaspoon oregano
1 teaspoon marjoram
Dash of salt and pepper

Preparation. Toast two slices of country white (or any) bread to deep brown and crush the bread in a bowl, then grind it to a powder in a chopper or blender. Melt butter in a saucepan, and pour over crumbs. Add tarragon, oregano, marjoram, and a dash of salt and pepper and stir to blend.

℀ *Apple and Acorn Squash Bake*

The sweet and spicy flavor of this blend is pure harmony and pleasure. It's perfect as it is, but there are two different seasonings you might try on individual servings: fennel or allspice. Dried, powdered fennel sprinkled on the hot dish gives the blend a greener nature. On another occasion, a dash of allspice will give the blend a deep, smoky richness. Serves 4.

1 medium acorn squash, skin on (or removed)

2 apples, peeled

¼ cup honey

2 teaspoons Dijon (or other brown mustard—not yellow)

3 tablespoons butter, melted

Preparation. Preheat oven to 350 degrees and butter a 9 × 13-inch baking dish. Cut acorn squash and apples into ½-inch slices. Combine honey and mustard. Arrange squash and apple slices in bottom of dish. Dot with butter. Drizzle honey-mustard sauce over top. Bake 45 minutes: Cover with foil for first ½ hour, and remove foil for last 15 minutes.

🌿 Beans and Ziti Casserole

The sauce is dark red, with a robust flavor that tastes like meat sauce, but it's pure vegetarian protein! A cinch to make! Tastes even better the next day. Try reheating a portion with ½ cup yogurt for a creamy flavor. For a variation, add 1 cup mixed vegetables, chopped.

3 cups ziti

2 cups ground plum or regular tomatoes (fresh or canned)

1 large can vegetarian baked beans (1 lb)

Herb Blend

1 teaspoon olive oil

2 teaspoons coriander

½ teaspoon cumin

2 teaspoons thyme

1 cup fresh parsley, chopped

Preparation. Cook ziti al dente, strain, return to saucepan, add tomatoes and beans, and blend. Add ingredients in Herb Blend and simmer for one minute. Ready to serve! For extra flavor, top servings with shredded Parmesan or cheddar.

🌿 Baked Eggplant and Cheddar Casserole

Cheddar adds a tangy taste to this eggplant casserole. Easy to make and easy to savor. Serves 4.

2 tablespoons butter
1 large, or 2 small eggplants
2 teaspoons dried oregano
2 pinches salt

Herbal Blend
1 cup onion, chopped
1 cup mushrooms, sliced
¼ cup fresh parsley, chopped
¼ cup bread crumbs
½ cup grated cheddar

Preparation. Grease casserole dish. Peel eggplant and slice it in slim rounds. Cut rounds in half. Drizzle 2 teaspoons of oregano and a dash of salt over the slices. Simmer eggplant in a saucepan with a small amount of water, until transparent and soft. Drain. Sauté Herbal Blend in butter until onions are transparent. Arrange in layers in casserole dish: a layer of eggplant topped with half of the Herbal Blend, followed by half of the bread crumbs, and half of the grated cheddar. Make a second layer with remaining eggplant, remaining Herbal Blend, remaining bread crumbs, and remaining cheddar. Bake at 350 degrees until the cheese melts and the bread crumbs are browned. Leftovers can be briefly reheated in the oven.

🌿 *Zesty Summer Squash Blend*

This spicy blend invigorates the mellow taste of summer squash, and it tastes even better the next day. This is a hearty amount, to give you leftovers for snacks and toppings.

- ½ cup chopped onion
- ½ cup sliced mushrooms
- 1 small, skinny hot or jalapeño pepper, chopped
- 2 tablespoons olive oil
- 8 cups summer squash, diced
- ⅓ cup tomato puree
- 2 teaspoons dried dill (or 4 teaspoons fresh)
- ¼ cup fresh parsley, chopped
- 2 cloves garlic, crushed
- ½ cup green olives with pimientos

Preparation. Sauté onion, mushrooms, and hot pepper in olive oil. Add squash and sauté for another minute. Add tomato puree, dill, parsley, and garlic. Stir well. Bring to a boil, reduce heat, and simmer for 15–20 minutes. Add green olives and pimientos and stir. Ready to serve! Chill half for the next day.

🌿 *Green and Dandy*

This double green blend gives you six dishes in one recipe. It features fresh dandelion leaves and your choice of one other green—asparagus, kale, collard, curly endive, Swiss chard, or spinach. You can make it with a different green each time, for six different varieties. The point is, you'll be getting the remarkable healing properties of dandelion leaves, which are a blood builder, digestive aid, and body cleanser to remove toxins, and they cool liver heat, which moves stagnant energy and lifts your mood. This combination uses collard greens. Serve warm.

2 cups dandelion leaves
2 cups collard greens
2 tablespoons olive oil
2 garlic cloves
1 teaspoon fresh lemon juice
Dash of salt and pepper to taste

Preparation. Lightly steam each green separately, keeping them a bit crisp. Chop greens into very small pieces in food processor or chopper. Heat olive oil in a skillet and lightly sauté garlic, add chopped greens, drizzle with lemon juice, salt, and pepper. Blend gently, and sauté on moderate heat for two to three minutes.

CHAPTER 15

Pasta and Rice Pleasure

✿ Saffron Rice

An exotic rice with a sweet, uplifting nature. To achieve a subtle blend, I chop the pistachios in small pieces and blend them into the rice like an herb. Saffron is best used sparingly, since too much saffron can overwhelm a dish. To gauge your saffron preference, begin by adding half of the saffron liquid to the rice, taste the rice, then add a little more saffron at a time, until you feel the saffron lift in the taste. Saffron rice enhances any meal, and it makes a luxurious snack. Take it to work in a plastic container for a lift. Tastes great hot or cold. With jasmine rice, the taste is subtle; with brown rice, it's hardy.

    3–4 strands of saffron
    1 cup white or brown rice
    ½ cup golden raisins
    ¼ cup pistachios, chopped fine
    1–2 teaspoons lemon pepper

Preparation. Place 3–4 strands of saffron in ¼ cup boiling water. Cover and set aside. Cook rice according to package instructions. For fluffy rice, turn off the heat under the rice just before all of the water is absorbed and keep the rice covered for a few minutes to absorb the rest of the water. (I like a dash of olive oil in rice to enrich the flavor.) Add raisins, pistachios, and 1 teaspoon of lemon pepper to the rice, then add the saffron liquid gradually and taste test to meet your saffron preference. If you want more zest, add the second teaspoon of lemon pepper. Note: The second time you make saffron rice, you will know your saffron preference, and you can add the strands directly to the water along with the rice. The saffron will infuse the rice as it cooks.

Turmeric Rice

Turmeric is commonly known as a spice in curry, but on its own, turmeric has a mellow nature with a hint of orange, and the antioxidant curcumin to fight Alzheimer's disease and cancer. It also helps to burn fat! This rice gives you turmeric in a gentle dish (not curried) that includes easy-to-digest protein from sesame seeds. Double the recipe and keep a supply on hand for snacks. Tastes great cold.

1 teaspoon turmeric
½ teaspoon grated fresh or dried ginger
1 teaspoon olive oil
1 cup white or brown rice
½ cup green pepper, chopped
½ medium onion, chopped
2 garlic cloves, chopped
4 teaspoons sesame seeds
Salt and pepper to taste

Preparation. Add turmeric, ginger, oil, and rice to boiling water. Cover rice and cook. Add chopped pepper, onion, and garlic to rice when it is fully cooked. Toast sesame seeds in a skillet without butter to golden brown, add to rice, and gently blend. Salt and pepper to taste. You can also make this rice without the sesame seeds, and you can vary the vegetables.

✌ Wild Rice with Roasted Red Pepper Puree and Shrimp

Black wild rice takes 50 minutes to cook, but it's worth the time. Make a pot full and refrigerate it for easy warming; add any *Magic Teaspoon* topping. Roasted Red Pepper Puree gives wild rice a sumptuous and penetrating flavor.

> 1 cup wild rice
> 1 cup whole shrimp, cooked
> ½ cup Roasted Red Pepper Puree (see chapter 8)

Preparation. Cook rice with a dash of salt according to package directions. Add shrimp to the warm rice, and stir in ½ cup of Roasted Red Pepper Puree.

✌ Sweet Veggie Stir Fry for Pasta or Rice

A light, refreshing blend that relies on the vegetables, herbs, and fruit for a mellow juice. Serve over delicate pasta like angel hair, or white rice like jasmine or basmati. Serves 2.

> 2 yellow peppers, sliced in strips
> 1 cup mushrooms, sliced
> 4 cloves garlic, diced
> 1 cup sweet Vidalia onion (or white), sliced in strips
> 2 teaspoons dried tarragon
> 2 teaspoons fresh or dried ginger
> 2 teaspoons olive oil
> ¼ cup golden raisins
> Optional: ¼ cup pineapple chunks or bits

Preparation. Sauté all ingredients except for pineapples and raisins in 2 teaspoons of olive oil until onion is transparent and blend is sizzling. Gradually add ¼ cup of water to create a sizzling juice. Blend in raisins and pineapples, and serve over pasta or rice.

Linguine al Pesto

Aromatic basil bliss! Play the music of the three tenors and savor the joy of making it. My friend Laura said that nothing beats going from her kitchen to her garden to pluck a handful of fresh basil for her Linguine al Pesto. Serves 2 generously.

Pesto
1 cup fresh basil leaves (press down tightly for measure)
1 clove garlic, crushed
1 tablespoon toasted pine nuts
¼ cup extra virgin olive oil
½ teaspoon salt
¼ cup fresh grated Parmesan
1 tablespoon fresh grated Romano
1½ tablespoons soft butter
2 medium tomatoes, peeled and seeded

½ pound linguini

Preparation. Pesto: Grind basil, garlic, pine nuts, olive oil, and salt in a food processor and transfer to a bowl. Add Parmesan and Romano by hand, and add butter. Dice tomatoes and set aside. Linguine: Cook linguine al dente in boiling, salted water. Before draining the linguine, remove 2 tablespoons of the cooking water and add it to the pesto, along with the chopped tomatoes. Spoon pesto over linguine, and blend well. Ready to serve!

✌ *Marinara Sauce for Any Pasta*

1 large can plum tomatoes (about 1 lb, 12 oz.)
1 small can tomato paste (8½ oz.), sugar free
2 cloves garlic, chopped
1 cup green pepper, chopped
1 cup onion, chopped
½ teaspoon oregano
½ teaspoon basil
¼ cup olive oil
¼ teaspoon pepper
Optional: 1 teaspoon sugar

Preparation. Set aside tomatoes and paste. Combine all other ingredients to yield a chunky mixture. Heat tomatoes and paste in a skillet, stir in vegetable blend, and bring to a boil. Reduce heat and simmer for 30–40 minutes minimum. The longer you simmer it, the better the blend gets. An authentic Italian blend simmers for several hours.

✌ *Poppy Seed Noodles with Peppers and Onion*

Poppy seeds have a calming nature and sweet, rich taste. You can use this for a vegetarian dish, with the pepper and onion topping. To turn it into a full-course meal with meat, nest a burger in the center of the poppy seed noodles with the chopped peppers and onions as a topping for the burger. That way, you can eat the poppy seed noodles plain (simply great), or blend the topping and burger bites into the noodles as you eat. Serves 2.

Herbal Topping
2 sweet red peppers, cut in strips (or 1 red and 1 orange)
2 small onions, cut in rings
2 cloves garlic, chopped
1 teaspoon lemon pepper
Salt and pepper to taste
2 teaspoons olive oil

2 cups thin, flat egg noodles
2 teaspoons poppy seeds
4 teaspoons butter

Preparation. Sauté Herbal Topping in 2 teaspoons olive oil until onion is transparent. A minute before you remove it from the heat, hit the blend with 2 teaspoons water to create juice. Cook noodles soft, and drain. In frying pan, toast poppy seeds in butter for 1–2 minutes. Pour over noodles and blend. Spoon Herbal Topping over noodles or nest in center.

Dinner Ease: Magic Teaspoon Pasta and Rice Versatility

Keep a selection of the *Magic Teaspoon* sauces, dips, and side dishes chilled, and high-energy eating is a cinch! All you have to do is make your favorite pasta or rice, and heat the topping. The salad dressings also make rich toppings for pasta and rice.

- Spaghetti with Rata-tat-a-touille (see chapter 14) or Great Green Sauce (see chapter 9) for a topping.

- Angel hair with Mediterranean Medley Vinaigrette or Green Goddess Dressing (see chapter 10) for a topping.

Any Veggie Crisp recipe (see chapter 12) can be used as a topping for pasta or rice. Make a two-cup portion and spoon it over your favorite rice or pasta. Quick and delicious dishes in a snap—filled with veggie vitality and herbal energy.

- Rice or pasta with Zucchini and Fennel Crisps.

- Rice or pasta with Eggplant and Thyme Crisps.

- Rice or pasta with Mexical Pepper Crisps.

You can also team up Veggie Crisps with sauces and purees for rice and pasta:

- Angel hair: Dill Deliverance puree (see chapter 8) in sour cream, topped with Onion and Turmeric Crisps.

- Spaghetti: Eggplant and Sesame Supreme (see chapter 9) topped with Two-Spice Pepper Crisps.

- Ziti: Black Bean and Corn Salsa (see chaper 9) topped with Mexical Pepper Crisps.

CHAPTER 16

Potatoes with Pizzazz

This international favorite is a natural for seasoning with herbs and spices. Filling and satisfying, the potato meets a modern herbal method for easy preparation with a garden of great herbs and spices for seasonings. They meet every expectation for pleasure and satisfaction.

Sizzling Red Bliss Side Dishes

In minutes, you can transform raw red bliss potatoes into fully cooked herbal blends. Use different herbs and spices each time you make the potatoes to accent lunches and dinners with a wide variety of herbal flavors. With this one recipe, you can make dozens of red bliss blends that taste like gourmet potatoes that you marinated for hours. I chose red bliss potatoes because they have a richer flavor than white potatoes, but you can also use white potatoes, sweet potatoes, or yams for these blends.

How to Make Sizzling Bliss Blends

Preheat oven to 500 degrees. You'll need a medium bowl that will fit 1 cup of diced potatoes comfortably. Cut potatoes in bite-sized pieces and place in bowl. Estimate 1 cup of potatoes per person. This recipe is based on 1 cup but can be increased easily.

> 1 teaspoon herb or spice of choice
> 4 teaspoons olive oil
> 1 cup red bliss potatoes, in bite-sized pieces

Preparation. Combine 1 teaspoon of herb or spice with 4 teaspoons olive oil. The mixture will be thick. Don't skimp on the herb—the full teaspoon gives you the rich flavor. Pour the blend over the potatoes in the bowl, and stir to blend thoroughly. Bake for 8–10 minutes. The potatoes will sizzle. Keep an eye on them the first time you make them, so you can gauge the time your oven takes to bake them thoroughly. Use a fork to test the softness the first time you make them. You can make two or three varieties at the same time to find your favorite, but each one has its own special taste.

CHILE–LEMON BLISS. Combine 1 teaspoon chile powder, 4 teaspoons olive oil, and 1 teaspoon fresh lemon juice for the blend.

ROSEMARY BLISS. Combine 1 teaspoon dried rosemary (or 2 teaspoons fresh, minced), 4 teaspoons olive oil, and ½ teaspoon lemon pepper for the blend.

THYME BLISS. Combine 1 teaspoon dried thyme (or 2 teaspoons fresh, minced) with 4 teaspoons olive oil for the blend.

DILL BLISS. Combine 1 teaspoon dried dill (or 2 teaspoons fresh, minced), 4 teaspoons olive oil, and ½ teaspoon lemon pepper for the blend.

SAGE BLISS. Combine 1 teaspoon dried sage (or 2 teaspoons fresh, minced), 4 teaspoons olive oil, and ½ teaspoon lemon pepper for the blend.

GARLIC BLISS. Combine 1 teaspoon dried garlic (or 2 teaspoons fresh, minced) and 4 teaspoons olive oil for the blend.

LEMON–PARSLEY BLISS. Combine 1 teaspoon dried parsley (or 2 teaspoons fresh, minced), 4 teaspoons olive oil, and ½ teaspoon fresh lemon juice for the blend.

CILANTRO AND GARLIC BLISS. Combine 1 teaspoon dried cilantro (or 2 teaspoons fresh, minced), ½ teaspoon garlic powder (or 1 teaspoon fresh, minced), and 4 teaspoons olive oil for the blend.

Healthy French Fries

Prepare the recipes above using the powdered or dried versions of the herbs and spices and cook the potatoes very crisp for French fries. Kids love them!

Savory Home Fries

Three traditional herbs give stove-top home fries a flavor to savor. Serves 2, based on one potato per person. This recipe is based on fresh potatoes with skins on, but you can use canned potatoes for convenience.

2 medium potatoes (or 1 large can, sliced)

Herbal Blend
1 cup chopped onions
1 teaspoon dried thyme
1 teaspoon dried rosemary
2 teaspoons fresh chopped parsley (or 1 teaspoon dried)
Salt and pepper to taste
2 teaspoons butter

Preparation. Cut potatoes—skins on—into small or large chunks. Cook in water until tender and drain. Sauté Herbal Blend in 2 teaspoons butter until onions are transparent. Add Herbal Blend to potatoes and gently fold in until potatoes are well coated. Cook over low heat, turning occasionally, until potatoes brown (15–20 minutes). If you prefer home fries that are more buttery, you can add additional butter as the potatoes brown.

Baked Potatoes and Yam Versatility

Top baked potatoes or baked yams with your favorite puree, sauce, dip, or Veggie Crisp recipe in *The Magic Teaspoon*.

- Baked potato or yam smothered with Dill Deliverance (see chapter 8) in sour cream.

- Baked potato or yam smothered with Zucchini and Fennel Crisps (see chapter 12) and a dollop of sour cream.

- Baked potato with whipped cottage cheese and Mexical Pepper Crisps (see chapter 12).

- Baked yam with Creamy Orange Nectar Dressing (see chapter 10).

- Baked potato smothered with Eggplant and Sesame Supreme (see chapter 9).

- Yam drenched in butter with Summer Squash and Sage Crisps (see chapter 12).

Mashed Potatoes and Mashed Yam Versatility

Mashed potatoes give you an opportunity to use your herbal butters with flair.

- Try mashed yams with Sage Butter (see chapter 6).
- Try mashed potatoes with Lemon–Parsley Butter (see chapter 6).

CHAPTER 17

Make a Little Magic with Chicken and Turkey

The secret for ease and versatility with chicken: One great recipe can take on an international air simply by changing the topping.

✿ *Mellow Ginger Chicken*

This golden chicken is subtle and sweet, tender and luxurious to eat. Make a large portion. When you reheat the chicken the next day, add a dash of water to the pan, and it will release a marvelous ginger sauce.

2 large boneless, skinless chicken breasts (double-sided)

2 cups sour cream

1 cup plain bread crumbs

4 teaspoons ginger

½ cup olive oil

Salt and pepper to taste

Preparation. Cut boneless chicken breasts into similar-sized pieces or strips. Set out two bowls. Put sour cream in one, and bread crumbs in the other. Add ginger to the sour cream and blend gently. Heat olive oil in a large frying pan. Dip each chicken chunk into the sour cream, followed by a dip into the bread crumbs, coating the chicken thoroughly. Sauté chicken in olive oil over low heat for 7–10 minutes on each side—the chicken will become a golden color on the outside. You will have more chicken than the pan allows in one sauté; therefore, remove the first round of chicken after 10 minutes, and sauté the second round. If you need more olive oil, use it freely. Return all of the chicken to the pan, cover, and cook over low heat for 15 minutes. If you prefer, you can salt and pepper the chicken before you begin for a zestier taste, or salt and pepper at the end, after a taste test. The chicken is supremely mellow without the added salt and pepper.

Mellow Ginger Chicken is one great recipe that can take any topping from simple to exotic. Transform it with any *Magic Teaspoon* topping.

- *Chicken Italian.* Top with Pesto with Pine Nuts (see chapter 9).

- *Tropical Island Chicken.* Top with Fresh Thousand Island Dressing (see chapter 10).

- *Mediterranean Chicken.* Top with Feta Cheese Dressing (see chapter 10).

- *Middle Eastern Chicken.* Top with Eggplant and Sesame Supreme (see chapter 9) or Red Pepper Puree (see chapter 8).

- *Tex-Mex Chicken.* Top with Fresh Salsa (see chapter 9).

- *Chicken in Bliss.* Top with Basil Bliss (see chapter 8).

- *All Dilled Up.* Top with Dill Deliverance (see chapter 8) in sour cream.

Imagine how easy it could be if you had a selection of fresh *Magic Teaspoon* sauces at your fingertips, in your refrigerator. Make a few sauces and dips at one time and store them in refrigerator bowls. All you have to do is remove one, heat, and top off any great chicken recipe.

Other great chicken recipes that can take on any topping:

- Broiled or grilled boneless chicken breasts: Baste with chopped fresh garlic, olive oil, and 1 teaspoon lemon pepper. If you like chicken with zest, add 1 teaspoon of chile powder to the basting blend.

- Chicken medallions: Cut chicken in 3-inch rounds and sauté in garlic and olive oil to brown. You can also buy the precooked medallions for quick herbal chicken with any topping.

Quick Chicken Cacciatore

A classic chicken dish with a rich, red sauce.

    2 boneless, skinless chicken breasts
    1 cup onion chunks
    4 cloves garlic, chopped
    ¼ cup chopped fresh parsley
    1 teaspoon Italian seasoning blend
    2 teaspoons olive oil
    1 medium can plum tomatoes (14–16 oz), peeled and seeded
    ¼ cup red wine vinegar
    1 cup green pepper chunks

Preparation. Lightly salt split chicken breasts. Brown onions, garlic, parsley, and Italian seasoning in olive oil. Add chicken and cook half way. Add tomatoes and red wine vinegar. Simmer for 5–10 minutes. Add peppers, and simmer until peppers are thoroughly cooked.

Rosemary Roaster and Rosemary Gravy*

1 whole chicken, 6–8 pounds
2 cloves garlic, minced
1 teaspoon thyme
2 teaspoons fresh rosemary, chopped (or 1 teaspoon dried, crushed)
¼ cup minced fresh parsley
2 teaspoons olive oil

Skin Baste
2 teaspoons butter, melted
1 teaspoon lemon pepper
Juice extender: 1 can low-salt chicken broth

*For variations: Substitute your favorite herb for the rosemary—marjoram, tarragon, sage, or peppermint.

Preparation. Preheat oven to 350 degrees. Wash chicken, dry with paper towels and put 2 minced garlic cloves and 1 teaspoon dried thyme in the cavity. Combine rosemary, parsley, and olive oil, and stuff half of blend under breast skin on each side. Combine butter and lemon pepper and baste skin with the blend. Bake chicken uncovered for ½ hour, then pour chicken broth over it. Baste twice until chicken is tender.

✌ *Roaster with Chile Powder Baste*

A simple but effective recipe. Use 1 teaspoon thyme, 2 cloves minced garlic, and ¼ cup chopped fresh parsley for cavity. Baste skin with 2 teaspoons butter and 1 teaspoon chile powder blended.

Make a Little Magic with Turkey

Remember: Spice Before You Salt

Don't be afraid to herb up your turkey. It will enhance the taste of the meat and gravy dramatically. Toss 2–4 cloves garlic, 2 teaspoons thyme, and 4 bay leaves into the cavity to enrich the taste of the gravy with powerful herbal energy. Don't add salt when you use lots of herbs—you don't need it.

Lift the breast skin and stuff Parsley Puree under the skin. **Parsley Puree:** 1 cup fresh parsley, 2 teaspoons fresh lemon juice, 2 cloves fresh garlic, and ⅛ cup extra virgin olive oil. Combine ingredients in a chopper and mince.

Bastes for the Skin

- Zest is best. Combine 2 teaspoons butter and 1 teaspoon of any zesty herb or spice—chile powder, paprika, or Rev It Up (see chapter 6).

- Any herbal honey makes an excellent baste for the skin of the turkey.

- Any herbal butter makes an excellent baste as well.

Use low-salt chicken broth as a juice extender, because the herbs will add so much flavor, salt isn't necessary. Cook the turkey with a foil tent and remove the foil a half hour before the turkey is done, to brown the skin.

If you don't stuff the cavity, use these stuffing variations:

- Stuff under the skin of the legs and breast—works beautifully, and the stuffing doesn't absorb all of the juices, as it often does in the cavity.

- Make small stuffing loaves (like small breads) or stuffing balls that are set in the cavity with room on the sides.

- Cook stuffing loaves in the oven in a separate pan (covered with foil), and baste the stuffing with pan juices every time you baste the turkey.

- Add lots of herbs to your stuffing and at least ½ cup chopped parsley.

CHAPTER 18

Make a Little Magic with Beef, Lamb, and Pork

The best way to incorporate beefy steaks and burgers into your menu is to limit them to three times a week, cooked well done. However, when you prepare beef with lots of vegetables, herbs, spices, and fillers, you can enjoy the rich taste of beef more often without overindulging because you're getting less beef in each serving.

Make Your Own Frozen Beef Entrees

When you are making beef recipes, take the opportunity to make frozen beef dinners that have all of the benefits of fresh beef meals, without additives or preservatives. Make hearty portions once, and freeze them for later use. I defrost fresh frozen beef dinners the easy way: place the frozen block in a skillet, add 1 cup water, and let it simmer to defrost and cook at the same time. Keep an eye on it, adding water as needed. You can turn a frozen dinner into a meal in about ten minutes.

🌿 Bay Leaf Beef with Gravy

The bay brings a deep, rich flavor to the beef and gravy, and baby portabella mushrooms are sumptuous with beef. This recipe gives you a generous amount, to have for leftovers or to freeze in portions for quick dinners.

    4 pounds London broil shoulder steak
    ¼ cup olive oil
    3 cloves garlic, chopped
    3 teaspoons dried thyme
    1 box (8 oz.) baby portabella mushrooms, sliced
    6 bay leaves
    Salt and pepper to taste

Preparation. Cut meat into bite-sized chunks and trim off all fat. Sauté meat in olive oil, garlic, and thyme in large pot until lightly browned on both sides. You will have to do two separate sautés to brown all of the meat, which shrinks as it cooks. Save the first round of meat and juices in a bowl, sauté second round, and combine both in the pot. Add 1½ cups water, portabella mushrooms, and bay leaves to the juices in the pot. Stir to blend. Salt and pepper to taste. Simmer for 2 hours. When meat is fork tender, make the gravy right in the pot with ¼ cup sifted flour stirred into the juices and blended. (Try brown wheat flour for extra richness.)

🌿 Thea Pota Pethilis's Greek Meatballs

This recipe has the perfect "hint" of mint—just a little—which is just enough to invigorate the herbal blend. The first time I made them,

I ate 8 meatballs right out of the pan. The second time I made them, I ate more than 8 meatballs right out of the pan. Let's just say, I should have doubled the recipe. They are delightful.

    2 pounds lean ground round
    2 tablespoons olive oil
    1 large onion, chopped fine
    4 slices bread
    2 eggs
    1 teaspoon oregano
    ½ teaspoon dried mint (or 1 teaspoon fresh)
    ¼ teaspoon pepper
    1 teaspoon parsley
    1½ teaspoons salt
    ½ cup thick tomato sauce

Preparation. Put meat in a bowl and set aside. To sauté the onion, start with a small amount of water and 1 tablespoon of olive oil in a large frying pan. Squash the onions as you sauté by pressing the onions down with a long-handled flat spatula to avoid splatter. Sauté until the water cooks away and the onion is soft. Add to meat. Soak the bread in water and squeeze it dry. Break the bread into small pieces and add to meat. Blend in the remaining ingredients and mix it together with your hands. Roll a tablespoon of mixture into a ball, coat with flour, and cook over medium heat in 1 tablespoon olive or vegetable oil until the meatballs are brown on all sides. Use extra oil if you need it.

❧ Shredded Carrot Meat Loaf with Dill

Shredded carrots and ketchup give this meatloaf a sweet flavor. Tastes even better the next day. I like to sauté the leftover slices in a frying pan to a toasty brown for a snack.

2 pounds ground round

1 medium onion, chopped (Vidalia or white)

¾ cup finely grated carrots (or shredded)

2 cloves garlic, chopped

2 teaspoons fresh dill (or 1 teaspoon dried)

¼ cup Fresh Ketchup* (or tomato paste)

Dash of olive oil

2 slices fresh bread

2 eggs, beaten

Dash of salt and pepper

*You can find the Fresh Ketchup recipe in Sugar Smarts (chapter 24).

Preparation. Preheat oven to 350 degrees. Place meat in a large bowl. Combine onion, carrots, garlic, dill, and ketchup in a food processor or chopper and mince. Soak the bread in water, and squeeze it dry. Break the bread into small pieces, and add to meat. Add eggs and carrot blend to meat, and salt and pepper. Blend by hand (thoroughly). Shape into a mound on a baking sheet or put in a meat loaf pan and bake for 1½ hours.

Fresh Bread Versatility for Your Meat Loaf

Fresh bread soaked in water and squeezed dry gives you a fresh, moist flavor in meat loaf that bread crumbs can't achieve. With fresh bread, you can vary the taste in the same meat loaf recipe simply by changing the bread you use and the onion you choose. I used sunflower–flax bread and Vidalia onion in one recipe for a light, sweet taste, pumpernickel and Bermuda onion in another. Sourdough and Vidalia onions give meat loaf a delicate taste, while dark rye and green onion give it zest. The versatility is fantastic; you can utilize the bread you have on hand to give every meat loaf its own special taste.

🌿 Meat Loaf Extravaganza

Extravagant herbs and spices give this high-energy meat loaf its rich flavor. You'll also find some unique fillers to choose from to keep life interesting. Make this meat loaf with ground buffalo or beef and bake in a narrow loaf pan.

    1 pound ground beef or buffalo
    ¼ cup finely chopped celery
    ¼ cup finely chopped onion
    ¼ cup chopped parsley
    1 tablespoon finely chopped fresh garlic
    2 tablespoons quality brown (not yellow) mustard
    ½ teaspoon salt
    ½ teaspoon black pepper
    1 teaspoon dried oregano
    2 teaspoons dried thyme
    1 egg
    ¼ cup chicken broth
    Filler of choice: ½ cup cooked rice, mashed potato, rolled oats, or
        bread crumbs

Preparation. Preheat oven to 350 degrees (325 degrees for a narrow loaf pan). Mash ground meat in a bowl. Add chopped celery, onion, parsley, garlic, mustard, salt, pepper, and dried herbs. Mix well. Break the egg into the blend, add broth, and mix well. Blend in ½ cup of your choice of fillers. Fill greased loaf pan with meat and smooth down. Cover and bake for 45 minutes. Let it cool for 15 minutes before serving.

🌿 *Ultra EZ Chili*

The secret ingredient that gives this chile a special flavor is cinnamon. You've got antioxidant power in this combination.

    1 pound ground beef
    ½ red onion, chopped
    3 cloves garlic, chopped
    1 teaspoon cumin
    1 teaspoon olive oil
    1 medium can red kidney beans (about 14 oz.), with juice
    1 medium can black beans (about 14 oz.), with juice
    1 small can chipotle chiles (6 oz. or 6–8 chiles)
    1 teaspoon chile powder
    ½ teaspoon cayenne pepper
    1 teaspoon cinnamon

Preparation. Sauté beef, onion, garlic, and cumin in olive oil. Add beans with juice and blend. Add chopped chiles, chile powder, cayenne, and cinnamon, and cook for 1 hour. Adjust hotness to taste with chile powder.

Burger for Dinner

A burger with herbal topping is an excellent dinner selection, served without a bun. Choose any *Magic Teaspoon* topping or puree for the burger, and top that with Onion and Turmeric Veggie Crisps for a touch of gold on your dinner plate. Mexical Pepper Crisps and Two-Spice Pepper Crisps are also excellent burger toppings, and you get your vegetables and meat in one step. (See chapter 12 for Veggie Crisps recipes.)

Make a Little Magic with Lamb Chops and Pork Chops

✌ *Grilled Stuffed Pork or Lamb Chops*

Preparation. Buy two thick pork chops or lamb chops and slice a pocket on the sides. Stuff the chops with any green puree—Basil Bliss, Garlic Whammo, Dill Deliverance (see chapter 8), or Parsley Puree (see chapter 5). Baste chops with butter, paprika, and garlic, or butter, chile powder, and garlic, or lemon pepper and garlic, or your favorite blend, and broil or grill.

✌ *Pear Pleasure Topping with Ginger–Mint Sauce*

Fruit toppings are a touch of luxury for pork and lamb chops. Estimate 1 pear half for each chop when you buy your canned pear halves. This recipe is for two chops.

    1 can of Bartlett pear halves (14–16 oz.)
    ½ cup pear juice from can
    ¼ teaspoon fresh mint, minced (or ⅛ teaspoon dried)
    ¼ teaspoon grated fresh ginger (or ⅛ teaspoon dried)

Preparation. Trim off bottom end of the pears to the match the length of the pork or lamb chops. Heat pear juice in a saucepan with mint and ginger. Place pear half on top of broiled chop, flat side down, and spoon the ginger–mint sauce over the top.

✒ *Apricot Puree Topping*

Use canned apricots to make a puree, and spoon the cool puree over hot pork or lamb chops. This is an ultra sweet topping.

    1 medium can apricots in juice (14–16 oz.)
    Dash of allspice

Preparation. Puree apricots (without juice) in a chopper or blender. If you want a smoother consistency, add a bit of the juice to the puree and blend to a creamy consistency. Spoon apricot puree over broiled pork or lamp chops and drizzle with a dash of allspice. You can vary this recipe by using mint instead of allspice.

✒ *Mango Slices and Mint*

Use fresh mango slices over pork or lamb chops, with a sprig of mint. Super sweet! You can also puree the mango slices in a chopper or blender and spoon it over the chops.

Creamy Sauces for Pork or Lamb Chops

Cinnamon Nectar, Creamy Orange Nectar Dressing, and Honey Yogurt Dressing make dreamy toppings for lamb or pork chops. Look for them in chapter 10.

CHAPTER 19

Make a Little Magic with Fish

✎ *Scallops So Simple and So Delicious*

This simple method for luxurious scallops can rise to any occasion in minutes.

    8 large scallops
    2 teaspoons fresh lemon juice
    1 teaspoon fresh parsley, minced
    ¼ cup of Mediterranean Medley Vinaigrette* (or your favorite bottled
        vinaigrette dressing)

*Find Mediterranean Medley Vinaigrette in chapter 10.

Preparation. Place scallops in a low-rimmed baking dish (2–3-inch-high edge). Drizzle lemon juice over the scallops, follow with parsley, and drizzle salad dressing over the top, letting an inch of the vinaigrette sit in the bottom of the dish. Bake in a toaster oven or regular oven at 375 degrees for 10 minutes or until the scallops are opaque. That's all there is to it! For an elegant fare, serve the scallops with avocado slices and Brie cheese with fresh rosemary pressed into the Brie.

Stir Fry Bay Scallops in Pesto Pasta

Total pleasure! For your sauce, use the recipe Pesto with Pine Nuts in chapter 9.

10–12 bay scallops
Dash of butter or olive oil
Linguine or other pasta cooked, al dente
Pesto with Pine Nuts recipe

Preparation. Rinse scallops and toss them into a frying pan with a dash of butter or olive oil on medium-high heat, and quickly cook for a few minutes until scallops are translucent, white, and firm. Add to pasta with pesto sauce.

Creamy Scallops Casserole

You can use your favorite herbs in the cream sauce to vary this recipe.

10 small or medium bay scallops
2 teaspoons lemon juice

Herbal Cream Sauce
2 tablespoons butter
3 tablespoons flour
1 cup milk
1 teaspoon quality mustard (or horseradish blend)
1 teaspoon dried tarragon

Preparation. Preheat oven to 375 degrees. Place scallops in small casserole dish. Drizzle with lemon juice. Cream sauce: Over low heat, melt butter in saucepan. Gradually drizzle flour into butter, whisking to blend. Gradually add milk, whisking to blend. Bring to a light boil, and whisk until sauce thickens (2 minutes). Turn off heat, and blend in mustard (or horseradish) and tarragon. Pour cream sauce over scallops and bake until tender (10 minutes).

White Fish Versatility

Drizzle any white fish with fresh lemon juice and sauté in 2 teaspoons olive oil and 1 clove garlic, chopped. (If you broil or grill, use the olive oil and garlic as a baste.) Choose your favorite *Magic Teaspoon* topping to turn plain white fish into a rich, herbal dish. You can also top white fish with fruit purees or Veggie Crisps.

- Great Green Sauce (see chapter 9).

- Basil Bliss or Dill Deliverance (see chapter 8) in ¼ cup yogurt and ¼ cup sour cream combined.

- Roasted Red Pepper Puree (see chapter 8) or Fresh Salsa (see chapter 9).

- Fresh Thousand Island Dressing (see chapter 10).

- Grilled pineapple with Onion and Turmeric Crisps (see chapter 12).

Salmon So Simple

Heat 2 teaspoons butter and 1 teaspoon dill, stirring to blend. Drizzle over salmon and grill or broil.

✿ Sole with Watercress and Almonds

Sauté sole in 1 teaspoon olive oil or butter and 1 clove garlic, crushed. Combine ¼ cup yogurt, ¼ cup sour cream, ¼ cup minced watercress, and 2–4 teaspoons chopped almonds for topping. If you would like the topping sweet, add ¼ teaspoon honey (or honey spread).

✿ Cold Shrimp with Fresh Cocktail Sauce

Use Roasted Red Pepper Puree for fresh cocktail sauce for your shrimp. See recipe in "High-Energy, High-Potency Herbal Purees" (chapter 8). You can also use Fresh Ketchup (see Sugar Smarts, chapter 24).

✿ Mussels in Saffron Sauce

Mussel lovers, rejoice!

    2 pounds mussels
    1 tablespoon extra virgin olive oil
    ¼ cup diced shallots
    2 cups dry white wine
    ⅛ teaspoon saffron (strands)
    2 tablespoons butter

    Bread for Dipping
    8 pieces of thick-sliced crusty bread
    2 teaspoons olive oil
    Salt and pepper

Preparation. Scrub mussels thoroughly. Preheat broiler. In a large stockpot over medium-high heat, combine olive oil and shallots and sauté until translucent. Add white wine and saffron and bring to a boil. When the liquid is boiling, add mussels, and cover pot. Cook for 6–8 minutes.

Bread: Brush both sides of bread with 2 tablespoons olive oil. Lightly salt and pepper each side. Broil the bread for a few minutes on each side until it is golden brown.

When the mussels are done, remove the mussels, and keep them warm in a bowl with aluminum foil cover. Bring the liquid in the pot to a boil again, and add the butter, whisking until melted. Pour the liquid over the mussels. Serve the toasted bread for dipping.

Mussels with Vermouth and Fennel

2 pounds mussels
1 large onion
¼ cup butter
½ cup vermouth
1 teaspoon fennel seeds

Preparation. Scrub mussels thoroughly. Sauté onion in butter until tender. Add mussels, vermouth, and fennel. Cover and steam until mussels open (3–5 minutes).

Feature: A Very Special Paella

Bill Bowman, who loves saffron, gave me his paella recipe to share with you, and wrote me a note about how this recipe came to be. I was so charmed by Bill's note, I wanted to share it with you, because it conveyed the very things that *The Magic Teaspoon* means to me— the magic of it all—life, the people we come to know, the ideas that inspire us, and the unique memories we carry with us—along with a recipe. This is what Bill wrote:

Like Obe Wan taught Luke, a master taught me paella. My English/ Irish roots never crossed with Spanish cuisine until my grandfather died, and a Spanish man offered my family his house on our cross-country journey to honor my grandfather. On the morning after the memorial service, I was instructed to fire up the paella pit with charcoal and logs. What happened over the next 6 hours revolutionized my cooking life.

The paella pit at his home was cut from earth and surrounded by large boulders for others to sit and watch the preparation. Every person around the pit enjoyed libations and were employed as cooks throughout the process. The saffron we used that day cost more than $100 an ounce. The pan was 4 feet in diameter. Needless to say, we used a lot of saffron.

Today, I cook my paella in a pan that is 2 feet in diameter, over charcoal with hickory chips. I also cook it stovetop in a smaller pan. Cooking is about the entire experience from planning the menu, to cooking it and serving it—letting others help, to share the experience.

✇ Paella—Seven Steps to Paradise

For your ease in making paella, the ingredients are listed in order of their appearance in the preparation of the paella. Where you see the dots . . . one step ends and the next step begins. If you take it step by step, it's a magical experience.

You'll need 2 cups of chicken broth divided into 1 cup portions (but keep some extra broth on hand). You'll also need a 10½-inch paella pan—a low, round pan with handles on each side (or you can use a large skillet)—1 small saucepan, 1 medium-sized bowl, and a roll of aluminum foil.

Have a paella party and let your company join in! Play music from Spain.

1

1 large boneless, skinless chicken breast, cut in bite-sized pieces

1 cup diced Sopressata dry sausage

1 tablespoon extra virgin olive oil . . .

2

1 small shallot, diced

1 large garlic clove, diced

1 medium tomato, diced

1 small onion, diced

1 pinch sweet paprika . . .

3

¼ teaspoon saffron threads

1 cup chicken broth . . .

4

1 cup medium-grain white rice

½ cup dry white Spanish wine . . .

5

1 cup chicken broth . . .

6

I pound littleneck clams, scrubbed . . .

7

½ pound uncooked shrimp, shell on, cleaned and deveined

(You might need the extra chicken broth here) . . .

Preparation.

Step 1. In a 10½-inch paella pan, heat olive oil on medium-high heat. Add the chicken and sausage, and sauté until ¾ cooked. Remove the meat mixture from the pan and keep it warm in a covered bowl.

Step 2. In the same pan, sauté the shallots, garlic, tomato, onion, and paprika, and cook it over medium heat until all of the liquid evaporates.

Step 3. Meanwhile, in a small saucepan, bring 1 cup of chicken broth to a boil. When it is boiling, turn off the heat and add the saffron threads to the liquid. Set aside.

Step 4. When the shallots–tomato blend has lost its liquid, add 1 cup of rice and stir, coating each grain of rice with the blend. Let it toast for 1 minute over medium-high heat. Then add the white wine and let the liquid cook until it is absorbed. Add the saffron–chicken broth, covering all of the rice, and turn the heat down to medium-low.

Step 5. After 10 minutes, add another cup of chicken broth and add the chicken–sausage blend to the pan, and stir.

Step 6. After 5 minutes, add the clams, nestling them into the bubbling broth. Cover the pan with foil and let it continue to cook.

Step 7. After 10 minutes, lift the foil and add the shrimp. You may need to add a little more chicken broth if the liquid has evaporated. Cover and cook for a final 5 minutes and turn off heat. Discard any clams that have not opened.

Serve the paella warm in the pan.

CHAPTER 20

Delectable
Soups to Savor

Soups are a fabulous resource for vegetable energy. Add herbs and spices, and you've got it all—energy, flavor and vitality, and lots of healing pleasure.

✶ *Absolute Broccoli Soup*

All broccoli, all luxury, and so simple to make, it's hard to believe. Broccoli has been found to help safeguard you from bladder cancer.

    1 head of broccoli florets
    2 teaspoons brown wheat flour
    4 teaspoons sour cream
    1 tablespoon half-and-half
    1 teaspoon lemon pepper or salt

Preparation. Use florets only; cut with a fraction of the stems on, and steam in water until tender. Transfer broccoli to a food processor or blender. Pour in 2 cups of water and blend on medium speed. Slowly add 2 teaspoons brown wheat flour to thicken and leave the top off the blender to let air penetrate the blend. Continue blending for 5 minutes until you get a thick green puree. If it looks chunky instead of creamy thick, gradually add a small amount of water to achieve creamy thickness. Transfer to a pot, and simmer for 10 minutes. You want a thick blend for this soup (not watery), so gradually add small amounts of water to the simmering puree until you reach a thick consistency you prefer. To cream the whole blend: add 4 teaspoons sour cream and 1 tablespoon half-and-half (you can add more if you want it creamier). Taste test and add salt, lemon pepper, or pepper if you want more zest. Serve it plain, or garnish with fresh grated Parmesan.

Curly Endive Soup

Rich in potassium, phosphorus, magnesium, calcium, iron, vitamins A and C—two of the ACE antioxidants for immunity and disease resistance—as well as protein and niacin. The best way to cut endive is with kitchen scissors.

    1½ cups curly endive
    ½ cup chopped onion
    3 cloves garlic, chopped
    1½ tablespoon butter
    1½ cups thick chicken broth
    1½ cups water
    Salt and pepper to taste

Preparation. Wash endive thoroughly and snip into ¼-inch pieces. Sauté onion and garlic in butter until onion is transparent. Add endive and sauté until wilted. Heat chicken broth and water in 2-quart saucepan. Add sautéed endive blend. Simmer for 15–20 minutes, until endive is soft. Add salt and pepper to taste. Serve soup hot, or chill and serve at your leisure.

🌿 *Pumpkin and Ginger Soup*

The renowned spice ginger gives this soup a warm nature, citrus gives it tang, and you receive antioxidant power.

    2 cups cooked pumpkin*
    2 cups chicken or vegetable broth
    2 cups milk (or soy milk)
    3 teaspoons minced fresh ginger
    ¼ cup orange juice concentrate
    Salt and pepper to taste

    *Winter squash can be used in place of pumpkin for a second great soup.

Preparation. Blend all ingredients on medium speed in a blender. Pour into a 2-quart pot and bring to a boil over high heat. Reduce heat and simmer for a half hour. Garnish with chopped fresh parley.

🌿 *Golden Carrot Soup*

A rich blend and a versatile soup that can be served warm in winter and cold in summer. It gives you everything from antioxidant power to immune system strength.

    6 medium carrots
    2 tablespoons chopped fresh ginger
    ¼ cup onion
    1 clove garlic, chopped
    2 tablespoons olive oil and 1 tablespoon butter
    1½ cups chicken broth* and 1½ cups water
    Salt and pepper to taste
    3 dashes of red pepper flakes

    *Vegetarians can substitute vegetable bouillon for chicken broth.

Preparation. Wash carrots and scrape off marks. Slice into slim rounds or strips. In a saucepan, sauté ginger, onion, and garlic in the olive oil and butter. Add carrots and briefly sauté to blend. Add chicken broth and water, salt and pepper flakes to taste, and hot pepper flakes. Bring to a boil, then reduce heat to simmer. Cover and cook until carrots are tender. Cool briefly, then process in blender until creamy (without lumps).

Serve immediately, or chill and reheat at serving time.

Note: If you prefer a mild version, omit the red pepper flakes.

✌ *Black Bean Soup with Cumin*

Deep and flavorful with spices galore! It's a whole-health tonic for spicy-soup lovers.

    1 large onion, chopped (1 cup)
    4 cloves garlic, finely chopped
    2 tablespoons vegetable oil
    1 pound dried black beans, picked over and rinsed
    2 cups cubed, precooked smoked ham
    6 cups chicken broth
    1 can (28 oz.) whole tomatoes with juice
    1 small can chipotle chiles (6 oz. or 6–8 chiles), diced
    2 tablespoons dried red chiles, diced
    2 tablespoons cilantro, chopped fine
    1 tablespoon oregano
    1 tablespoon cumin

Preparation. Cook onion and garlic in vegetable oil over medium heat, stirring frequently until onion is tender. Add black beans, ham, chicken broth, tomatoes with juice, chipotle chiles, diced red chiles, cilantro, oregano, and cumin. Bring to a boil, lower heat, cover, and simmer until beans are tender—about 2 hours. Now you're going to puree it in two batches. Pour 3 cups of soup into a blender and whirl until smooth. Transfer to pot and blend remaining soup.

🌿 Leeks and Asparagus Soup

Asparagus lovers, there's tarragon and onion flavor to thrill you, along with powerful health benefits.

2 bunches asparagus

1 leek, diced

1 medium onion, diced

1 teaspoon tarragon

2 tablespoons olive oil

1 cup milk (or soy milk)

1 cup chicken broth

Salt and pepper to taste

Preparation. Cook asparagus in water until tender, and drain. Sauté leek, onion, and tarragon in olive oil until onion and leek are translucent. Blend asparagus and leek–onion mixture in blender at medium speed. Slowly add milk, followed by chicken broth. Transfer to pot. Use extra milk and chicken broth in equal parts until you reach the consistency you desire. Taste test first, salt and pepper afterward. Heat and serve.

🌿 Curly Kale Soup

Kale is low in fat, calories, and sodium, with rich antioxidant power for cancer fighting and disease resistance.

2 cups curly kale

2 cups vegetable bouillon

4 tablespoons chopped onion

2 teaspoons chopped garlic*

2 tablespoons olive oil*

2 heaping teaspoons fresh miso paste

*If you increase the volume of this recipe, use no more than 3 cloves of garlic, and no more than 4 tablespoons of olive oil.

Preparation. Steam kale leaves in bouillon until tender—about 10 minutes. Leave kale in bouillon. Sauté onion and garlic in 2 teaspoons olive oil until transparent, then transfer to blender. Add miso. Remove kale from bouillon and add to blender, using some of the bouillon to process the kale thoroughly. Blend until the mixture is smooth. Return it to the pot with the remaining bouillon and stir well. Ready to serve.

Feature: One Great Chicken Soup Is All You Need

Chicken soup is a time-honored cure-all. Speculation about the curative nature of chicken soup has continued through the ages. What could it be that makes this soup so special? Herbs! Every ingredient, except the chicken, is an herb, even the ones that are commonly called vegetables—onions, parsnips, carrots, and celery. This recipe was given to me by a friend, who got it from her grandmother. This is Yetta's recipe. It's a classic.

✿ *Grandma Yetta's Chicken Soup*

1 chicken (whole, or cut into parts)
1 parsnip, peeled, ends removed
4 large carrots, peeled, ends removed
1 onion, ends removed
1 whole bunch of celery, leaves on
2 bay leaves
¼ cup chopped fresh parsley
Salt and pepper to taste

Preparation. Cover chicken with water in a large saucepan—skin on. (If you want a low-fat broth, remove the skin, or remove half of the skin for a midpoint.) Cut parsnips and 2 carrots lengthwise in strips and add to water. Set the other 2 carrots aside. Cut onion in half and add to water. Remove stalks from celery, cut off bottom, and chop hearts of celery, including leaves from tops of stalks, and add celery to the water. Add parsley and bay to the water. Bring to a boil, reduce heat, cover, and simmer for 40–60 minutes, until chicken is tender. Remove chicken and bones from broth and set aside to cool.

Broth: Strain broth though a sieve. Discard vegetables (their nutrients are depleted). Return broth to saucepan. Cut the 2 fresh carrots in slim strips and sauté until tender. Add to broth. Add half of the chicken pieces to broth. Taste test and add salt and pepper to preference. The broth is now ready! (Use the leftover chicken for a Casual Cold Burrito Platter—see chapter 13.)

Noodles or Matzo Balls

EGG NOODLES. If you add thin egg noodles to your chicken broth, cook them on the side and add them to the warm broth each time you serve the soup to keep the noodles from becoming soggy.

MATZO BALLS. If you add matzo balls to your chicken broth, cook them on the side and add them to the broth before serving, since matzo balls can soak up the broth if they are refrigerated in the broth. For instance, you can refrigerate the broth with 5 matzo balls, and the next morning, you'll have 5 "souped-up" matzo balls and no broth. Matzo balls often need to be cooked longer than the package directions indicate if you don't want undercooked matzo balls, called *sinkers.* You want floaters, which are cooked longer to become light.

CHAPTER 21

Desserts from Cool to Sweet

Rely on fresh fruit energy for your desserts, and you'll get plenty of sweetness in a healthy package, with fiber, vitamins, minerals, and the vital energy of herbs and spices for a boost of healing pleasure.

❧ *Sweet Banana Rapture*

Fried bananas with a sweet, nutty flavor and sour cream topping. Takes minutes to prepare! You don't need plantain bananas, plain are perfect! Plan on one banana per person. For each serving:

> 2 teaspoons sesame seeds
> 1 banana, sliced lengthwise and halved (4 thick pieces)

Preparation. Sauté sesame seeds to a toasty, golden brown in a frying pan (you don't need butter—heat releases oil in the seeds). Add bananas to toasted sesame seeds, and flip over to coat both sides. Fry both sides of bananas for 1 minute. Serve slices warm with a dollop of sour cream.

✽ *Pear Paradise*

These pears are drizzled with ginger–mint sauce and topped with dessert whip. Use canned pears and save the juice. Serves 2, based on 2 pear halves per person.

½ cup pear juice from can
¼ teaspoon fresh ginger
¼ teaspoon dried mint (or ½ teaspoon fresh)
4 pear halves
¼ cup dessert whip

Preparation. Heat pear juice in a small saucepan. Add ginger and mint and blend for about 30 seconds while simmering. Spoon the warm sauce over the pear halves and top with a dollop of dessert whip. For a chic presentation, serve the pear slices on cobalt-blue plates.

Creamy Fruit Parfaits

The candy colors of these creamy parfaits are as tempting as their tastes. They only take a few minutes to make, but no one would believe they didn't take hours. You can use fat-free yogurt, low-fat sour cream, and fat-free dessert whip without sacrificing richness. Serve the parfaits plain or fancy, with chopped nuts as a topping. Make them in multiple colors for a special dinner or party, served in stemmed glass dishes. You can also make rainbow parfaits, layering the colors with chopped nuts between the layers. It's a wonderful way to get the health benefits of fruits in your everyday menu.

✌ *Creamy Apricot Parfait*

1 can apricots (15 oz.), drained of juice
¼ banana
¼ cup sour cream
¼ cup yogurt
3 teaspoons dessert whip

Preparation. Puree apricots and banana in small chopper or blender. Add sour cream and yogurt, and blend. Add dessert whip, and blend. Use glass dessert dishes to display the creamy apricot color. Chill.

CREAMY ORANGE PARFAIT. Follow the directions for Creamy Apricot Parfait but substitute one 15 oz. can of mandarin orange segments, drained of juice, for the apricots.

CREAMY PEACH PARFAIT. Follow the directions for Creamy Apricot Parfait but substitute one 15 oz. can of peaches, drained of juice, for the apricots.

CREAMY PAPAYA PARFAIT. Follow the directions for Creamy Apricot Parfait but substitute 1 medium papaya for the apricots. Also add 3 cherries to the blend.

CREAMY MANGO PARFAIT. Follow the directions for Creamy Apricot Parfait but substitute pulp of 2 fresh mangoes for the apricots.

CREAMY STRAWBERRY PARFAIT. Follow the directions for Creamy Apricot Parfait but substitute 2 cups of frozen strawberries, thawed, for the apricots. Increase the sour cream and yogurt to ½ cup each. Use extra strawberries if you want it thicker. Add a dash of allspice and a dash of vanilla to the blend.

Swedish Peppernuts

Peppernuts are Swedish shortbread cookies made in small, round balls. Three great spices charm these cookies: cinnamon, cardamom, and white pepper. It's a Swedish tradition to make them as holiday gifts, and it's a great activity to do with children, who love to roll the balls, and love to eat them. This recipe makes 50 small cookies, but you might want to double it, because you'll have to hide them if you want to keep them around. If you make them for holiday gifts, bake them a few weeks ahead and store them in tins. The spicy flavor gets even richer with time.

¼ pound of butter, softened	½ teaspoon baking soda
½ cup sugar	1 teaspoon cinnamon
¼ cup heavy cream	½ teaspoon cardamom
2 cups all-purpose flour	½ teaspoon white pepper
¼ teaspoon baking powder	

Preparation. Preheat oven to 350 degrees. Cream butter and sugar together. Stir in cream. Sift dry ingredients and add to the butter mixture. Mix together with your fingertips until you have soft dough that sticks together. Chill 15 minutes. Form the dough into balls the size of marbles. Place them on a cookie sheet and bake for 16 minutes.

California Trifle

A star in the roster of rich desserts, with strawberries and cream, kissed by almond and garnished with mint. Serve in a glass compote bowl (or any glass bowl on a pedestal) 10–12 inches in diameter.

1 cup milk
1 box vanilla instant pudding
1 cup heavy cream, whipped
2 teaspoons almond extract
2 packages lady fingers
2 cups fresh strawberries (or frozen, thawed), crushed
½ cup fresh mint leaves for garnish

Preparation. Use only 1 cup of milk to make a thick pudding. Whip cream separately and gently fold it into the pudding with the almond extract. Refrigerate 10 minutes. Line the bottom of a dessert dish with ladyfingers. Drizzle with juice from strawberries. Layer with pudding blend, followed by crushed strawberries, another layer of pudding, and a top layer of strawberries. Garnish with fresh mint leaves. Chill. (Note: Thawed frozen strawberries will give you a rich juice, which you might prefer for this dessert. To get juice from fresh strawberries, add water as you crush them, to create the juice.)

℘ *Peachy Keen Tapioca*

Ginger, mint, and vanilla transform tapioca pudding into a rich pudding or sauce to spoon over sliced fruit, or create a layered dessert with tapioca between the layers of fruit. This blend will give you many fruit desserts; make it with pear slices, kiwi slices, mango slices, sliced strawberries, sliced bananas, or a combination. Simply substitute your favorite fruit for the peaches in the recipe.

1 box tapioca pudding
½ teaspoon fresh or dried ginger
½ teaspoon dried mint (or 1 teaspoon fresh)
Dash of pure vanilla extract
4 halves fresh peaches, or canned (drained of juice)

Preparation. Cook tapioca pudding according to package directions and transfer to blender. Add ginger, mint, and vanilla, and whip.

Layered Dessert: Slice peaches into small pieces. Begin with tapioca on bottom layer, follow with peaches, tapioca, peaches, and tapioca. Top with mint leaf or cherry.

✿ Saucy Apples

This dessert gives you individual apple pies that bake in 8–10 minutes. You have to make these apples to believe the taste. To serve, spoon apples over dessert shells with a dollop of dessert whip, which will melt into the hot apples. They also taste great chilled. Serves 4–6.

   4 apples, peeled and sliced
   ¼ cup golden raisins
   ¼ cup chopped walnuts
   ½ teaspoon nutmeg
   ⅓ cup water
   1 or 2 teaspoons honey
   1 teaspoon pure vanilla extract

Preparation. Preheat oven to 350 degrees. Combine all ingredients except vanilla in a casserole dish with the water in the bottom of the dish. Bake 8–10 minutes, or until apples are transparent and begin to soften but still have their shape (you don't want applesauce). Remove from heat and gently blend in vanilla. Ready to serve. Note: If you like very sweet apples, use 2 teaspoons honey, less sweet, use 1 teaspoon. I usually use 1 teaspoon.

🌿 *Fruit Cup with Cinnamon Nectar Topping*

The best three-fruit combinations to use with this spectacular topping are:

- Green grapes, sliced bananas, and blueberries

- Sliced apricots, bananas, and raspberries

- Peaches, pears, and blueberries

Cinnamon Nectar Topping: Blend ¼ cup sour cream, ¼ cup yogurt, ¼ teaspoon honey, and ¼ teaspoon cinnamon. Serve over fruit in a glass dessert bowl, or layer the fruits with chopped nuts and Cinnamon Nectar Topping in a stemmed glass dessert dish to highlight the colors of the fruits.

CHAPTER 22

Magic Teaspoon Iced Teas

Ten Power Drinks for Your Healing Pleasure

A healthy menu isn't complete without healing teas.

I've taken iced teas to a new level for pleasure and energy in these signature teas that use herbs, spices, and fruits to boost their healing power. They can be a powerful resource for your immunity and well-being to fight many major diseases and to lift your spirits. They even provide body fat reduction. They come to you with my blessings to be the best that you can be.

Health profiles for the herbs in these teas can be found after the iced tea recipes. That way you can get right to the recipes, then read up on the herbs while your tea is chilling. For health profiles of the spices used in these teas, visit chapter 2, "Nature's Bouquet of Healing Herbs and Spices for Cooking."

The herbs for these teas were chosen for their wholesome natures, all-inclusive healing power, versatility, and strength. They will give you some very valuable herbs that you might not use routinely as hot teas—herbs that are vital resources for natural healing. You'll notice how good they make you feel with the first glass.

These iced teas can also help you cut excess sugar from your body by using one or two teas to replace colas or sugary fruit drinks each day. See chapter 24, "Sugar Smarts," to discover how many teaspoons of sugar you can remove from your system in one week.

What Can You Use for a Sweetener?

I drink these teas without added sweeteners, relying on the natural flavor that the herbs, spices, and fruits provide. However, many people prefer extra sweeteners in teas, and if that's the case for you, what should you do?

Stevia: A Natural Gift of Sweetness and Zero Sugar

Stevia is a healthy herb that provides rich, natural sweetness without sugar. It comes from the leaves of the herb *Stevia rebaudiana*, a native to Brazil and Paraguay. It's 300 times sweeter than sugar, with a refreshing, sweet taste, and a little goes a long way. It can be a valuable aid for people with diabetes to help to reduce your blood sugar level without sacrificing sweetness! It's also great for dieters to feed sugar cravings without using sugar, and stevia is low in calories. Stevia contains vital nutrients, including magnesium, potassium, phosphorus, manganese, selenium, silicon, sodium, calcium, iron, and zinc. This herb with natural sweetness is used in South America to treat diabetes and hypertension. Stevia is available in packets, but it also comes in a dropper bottle that is easy to use and portable. The drops can be added to any drink to make your measurements a cinch. Use the following formula to use stevia instead of sugar: 2 drops stevia equals 1 teaspoon sugar.

Honey: Natural Sugar
with Stable Absorption

Honey is absorbed slowly, which has a more stable effect on blood sugar than does white sugar or corn syrup sugars. Slower absorption means more energy over a longer term, and it's often used by athletes for endurance sports. Honey is antibacterial to fight infections, it helps to speed healing and recovery, and it contains micronutrients including citric and amino acids, enzymes, B-complex, folic acid, vitamin C, magnesium, calcium, sodium, silicon, chlorine, copper, sulfur, and iron. It has a calming nature to fight stress and ease insomnia and has a reputation for improving immunity. Scientists are researching the micronutrients in honey, which they believe may have very significant benefits for health and disease prevention. It has been used to treat cardiovascular disease and indigestion, and it's a time-honored treatment to speed healing, fight colds, allergies, and respiratory conditions. If you use honey to fight allergies, your best bet is to buy locally harvested honey, which will help to desensitize you to the effects of pollen that is particular to your area.

The Eternal Spring: Water

One of the most important benefits of iced teas is something we take for granted, and yet it's the most important drink for your health: water. One pitcher of an iced tea gives you four glasses of water, half of the recommended dose of water for each day. Water is vital for every process from fat reduction to healthy brain function. It's a natural appetite suppressant, it helps to metabolize fats and reduce fat deposits in your body, it's the best treatment for water retention, it cleanses the body of excess salt, and it maintains healthy muscle tone and firm skin. Water is a must for a healthy heart, it prevents constipation and balances body fluids, and it's essential to fight diseases, because it cleanses the body of wastes and toxins. Every system in your body needs water to function properly. It's essential for the absorption and assimilation of nutrients.

Water is also the best method to get the most reliable benefits from herbs and spices. It delivers the health properties from herbs and spices to your body in a manner that is harmonious with your body's natural processes. Unlike capsules, herbs and spices in water follow the natural course of digestion from your mouth through your system, which is an automatic regulator for substances that enter your body.

Could it get any easier to get the water you need, with healing benefits and satisfaction as part of the drink?

🌿 Green Tea Sunrise

This is the way to invigorate your day. Every ingredient has healing benefits. Green tea is a circulatory tonic with antioxidants that help to fight cancer; it's antidiabetic, antiaging, and heart smart; and studies show that people who drink green tea regularly have 10 percent less body fat than non–tea drinkers. Fennel is a natural antacid, anti-inflammatory, rich in nutrients, and it helps to keep you lean. Coriander lifts your spirits, helps to reduce blood sugar levels, lowers cholesterol, and eases tension. Carry Green Tea Sunrise in a thermos to work.

    4 bags green tea
    1 teaspoon dried coriander
    2 teaspoons dried fennel
    Juice of ½ orange
    Juice of ½ lemon
    Optional: 1 teaspoon honey or 2 drops of stevia

Preparation. Boil 3 cups of water in a small saucepan. When it reaches a boil, turn off heat, add green tea bags, and let them steep for 5–8 minutes. Add coriander and fennel, and let the tea sit for another minute. Transfer to a tall pitcher (about 2 quarts), add orange and lemon juice, fill the pitcher with water and ice, and chill.

🌿 *Green Tea and Turmeric Gold*

I'm excited about this iced tea. It's a one-two punch to help to fight cancer. This tea combines two antioxidant compounds—found in green tea and turmeric—which research shows have a synergistic effect to prevent or inhibit the growth of cancer cells. (See sidebar for more details.) I used powdered turmeric for this tea, which turns the water to liquid gold. Turmeric is a sacred root in India. It also fights diabetes, it's a natural anti-inflammatory, and it's good for your heart. Researchers also suggest that turmeric may work better with a little fat, so the best time to take this tea is during meals or after you've eaten and have some fat to digest.

> 4 bags decaffeinated green tea
> 1 teaspoon turmeric (powdered root)
> 1 small can (or 1 cup) mandarin orange segments
> Optional: 1 teaspoon honey or 2 drops of stevia to sweeten

Preparation. Boil 3 cups of water in a small saucepan. When it reaches a boil, turn off heat, add green tea bags, and steep for 5–8 minutes. Remove tea bags and add turmeric. The water will turn gold. Let it steep for another minute, stirring to blend it. Transfer to a tall pitcher (about 2 quarts). Puree orange in chopper or blender, add puree to pitcher, fill with water and ice. Chill. Taste test it chilled before you sweeten.

ONE-TWO PUNCH TO HELP FIGHT CANCER

Recent studies have revealed that a compound in green tea (epigallo-catechin-3-gallate) and a compound in turmeric (curcumin) have the ability to prevent and inhibit the growth of cancer cells. In an in vitro study of these compounds and their effect on oral cancers, catechins in green tea showed anticarcinogenic effects on cell lines tested, along with anti-inflammatory and antioxidant effects. Curcumin in turmeric also showed anticarcinogenic effects on cell lines tested. Several cell lines were tested, and both green tea and turmeric demonstrated the ability to inhibit cancer cell growth in all cell lines that were tested.

Synergistic activities were also noticed when both compounds were used: green tea's catechin, epigallocatechin-3-gallate, and turmeric's curcumin. By using the two compounds together, researchers were able to achieve the same results while the dosage of each was reduced. It's called a one-two punch, and it helps to fight cancer.

✌ Astragalus Mint Tonic

Powerful health protection makes this iced tea special. Astragalus is known as the immunity root in China, an herb that boosts immunity, fights infections, helps to fight heart disease, and comes packed with nutrients for stamina and health. Mint (spearmint or peppermint) is a tonic herb with flavonoids to fight many major diseases; it's a natural decongestant, pain reliever, and a digestive aid; and it eases stress and tension.

4 bags astragalus tea

2 bags mint tea (spearmint or peppermint)

1 small can (or 1 cup) pineapple chunks (or crushed)

Juice of ½ orange

Optional: 1 teaspoon honey or 2 drops of stevia to sweeten

Preparation. Boil 3 cups water in a small saucepan. When it reaches a boil, turn off heat, add teas, and steep for 5–8 minutes. Remove from heat, transfer to a tall pitcher (about 2 quarts). Puree pineapples in a chopper or blender, add the puree and orange juice to the pitcher, fill with water, and chill. Strain the drink to remove the pineapple pulp after it chills for a deep pineapple flavor. Taste test chilled before you sweeten.

✿ Rose Hips Tonic Tea

Rose hips make a vibrant red tonic for mental clarity and full-body health. It's an excellent antiaging iced tea that provides protection from disease, tones the organs, promotes faster healing, is a calmer nature, and everything in between. Mint is known as a cure-all and calming herb, and coriander is a spirit lifter and vitality spice that also eases tension.

> 4 bags rose hips tea
> 2 bags mint tea (I use spearmint)
> 1 teaspoon coriander
> 1 cup frozen strawberries, pureed
> Juice from ½ orange
> Optional: 1 teaspoon honey or 2 drops of stevia to sweeten

Preparation. Boil 3 cups of water in a small saucepan, turn off heat, add rose hips and mint tea bags, cover, and let it steep for 5–8 minutes. Remove tea bags, add coriander, and steep for one minute. Puree 1 cup thawed frozen strawberries with juice in a chopper or blender. Transfer tea to a tall pitcher (about 2 quarts), add strawberries, orange juice, and fill with water and ice. Chill. You can strain the drink when it is chilled or drink it with the strawberry pulp, like I do. Taste test chilled before you sweeten.

🌿 *Saffron Holiday*

A spirit-lifting tea and tonic for the body and mind, with saffron, considered a rejuvenating spice. Three great herbs harmonize with saffron for maximum energy: rose hips, cranberry, and mint. Float lime and orange slices on top.

> 3 threads saffron
> 2 bags rose hips tea
> 1 bag cranberry tea
> 1 bag mint tea
> Optional: 1 teaspoon honey or 2 drops of stevia to sweeten

Preparation. Saffron yields its properties to boiling water, but it can take a while, so start the saffron before you start to make the tea. Place saffron threads in ¼ cup boiling water, cover, and set aside. To make the tea, boil 3 cups of water in a small saucepan, add rose hips, cranberry, and mint tea bags, and steep for 5–8 minutes. Remove tea bags, transfer to a tall pitcher (about 2 quarts), and add saffron water. If some of the threads have not dissolved, remove them. Fill the pitcher with water and ice. Chill. Taste test chilled before you sweeten.

🌿 *Saffron Holiday Punch*

Increase the volume of Saffron Holiday iced tea, and puree extra fruits to sweeten the blend. Try strawberries, oranges, and mangoes for one puree; pineapples, oranges, and papayas for another. Float pineapple bits, orange slices, strawberry slices, and lime slices on top. Serve it at your next party or gathering of friends.

🌿 Elderberry Tonic Tea

Elderberry is a proven flu fighter and respiratory remedy for colds, hay fever, allergies, and mucous conditions. I've added feverfew to this blend, because it's a natural antihistamine. High histamine production has been linked to allergies, hay fever, and headaches. This is the blend to reach for to strengthen the breath of life.

6 bags elderberry tea
1 bag feverfew tea
1 cup frozen blueberries
Juice of ½ fresh lemon
Optional: 1 teaspoon honey or 2 drops of stevia to sweeten

Preparation. Boil 3 cups of water in a small saucepan. When it reaches a boil, turn off heat, add tea bags, and steep for 5–8 minutes. Transfer to a tall pitcher (about 2 quarts). Puree frozen blueberries in juice. Add blueberries and lemon juice to pitcher. Fill with water and ice. Chill. Taste test chilled. Blueberries can be tart—add honey if you want it sweeter.

🌿 Vibrancy Tonic for Women

This blend is a vital energy tonic for both sexes, but particularly for women. Three vivid herbs combine for hormone balance, harmony, and antioxidant protection from cell damage and premature aging. Astragalus is an immune system booster, a vital energy tonic, and a balancing herb. Dong quai is a chi tonic, a balancing herb for hormones, good for PMS tension and menopausal vitality, with no estrogenic properties. It's a circulatory tonic to enhance concentration and memory, maintain a healthy heart, and help to build bone marrow to fight osteoporosis. Cranberry is the E. coli fighter with antioxidants, vital for healthy kidneys, bladder, and urinary tract.

> 1 bag astragalus tea
> 2 bags dong quai tea
> 2 bags cranberry tea
> 1 small can (or 1 cup) mandarin orange segments
> Optional: 1 teaspoon honey or 2 drops of stevia to sweeten

Preparation: Boil 3 cups of water in a small saucepan. When it reaches a boil, turn off heat, add tea bags, and steep for 5–8 minutes. Transfer to a tall pitcher (about 2 quarts). Puree mandarin orange segments, using a dash of the syrup to create a smooth puree. Add orange puree to pitcher, and fill with water and ice. Chill. (If you don't want the orange pulp in your drink, press the puree through a strainer and use only the juice.) Experiment with your favorite fruits as purees to vary this blend. Taste test chilled before you sweeten.

✌ *Raz-a-ma-taz*

For immune insurance and heart health, to fight inflammation and keep E. coli off your bladder walls, this rich blend gives you everything and something extra. Milk thistle tea contains silymarin, a combination of flavonolignans that have the unique ability to bind toxins in the body before they can reach the liver. It renews liver energy, which has a beneficial effect on every system of your body, even your mood. Milk thistle fights depression.

> 1 bag milk thistle tea
> 4 bags cranberry tea
> 2 bags astragalus tea
>
> 1 cup frozen raspberries, thawed
> 1 cup frozen strawberries, thawed
> Optional: 1 teaspoon honey or
>   2 drops of stevia to sweeten

Preparation. Boil 3 cups of water in a small saucepan. When it reaches a boil, turn off heat, add tea bags, and steep for 5–8 minutes. Transfer to a tall pitcher (about 2 quarts). Puree raspberries and strawberries in a chopper or blender and add to pitcher. Fill with water and ice. Chill. Taste test chilled before you sweeten.

Orange Sunset

Orange and chamomile give this iced tea an ultrasweet harmony. The blend eases tension, fights insomnia, and has lots of antioxidant power to fight free radical damage, and chamomile is a powerful anti-inflammatory to fight all inflammatory diseases.

> 4 bags chamomile tea
> 1 small can (or 1 cup) mandarin orange segments
> Optional: 1 teaspoon honey or 2 drops of stevia to sweeten

Preparation. Boil 3 cups of water in a small saucepan. When it reaches a boil, turn off heat, add tea bags, and steep for 5–8 minutes. Transfer to a tall pitcher (about 2 quarts). Puree mandarin oranges in a dash of their syrup for a smooth blend. Add puree to pitcher. Fill with water and ice. Chill. Taste test chilled before you sweeten.

Herbal Garden for the
Magic Teaspoon Iced Teas

ASTRAGALUS

Astragalus membranaceus
PART USED: **Root**

Known as the immunity root, this sweet-natured white root from China and Mongolia is a member of the pea family, with deep, medicinal roots. It's an immune system booster that strengthens white blood cells and stimulates the production of antibodies and interferon to fight diseases, including cancer. It's antiviral and antimicrobial, and it helps to renew the adrenal glands—excellent for fatigue, exhaustion, and recovery from illness. It's a health protector with amino acids, polysaccharides, linoleic acid, betaine, choline, and glycosides, and it's a circulatory tonic to strengthen the cardiovascular system, improve brain function, help reduce high blood pressure, and balance body fluids.

CHAMOMILE

Chamaemelum nobile (Roman Chamomile),
Matricaria chamomilla (German Chamomile)
PART USED: **Flowers**

Called the comforter, this mellow floral herb is a natural tranquilizer, one of the nine sacred herbs of the Saxons. It's a natural anti-inflammatory to ease aches, pains, and cramps, excellent for the aches and pains of arthritis and any inflammatory disease (diseases that end in *itis*—tendonitis, gastritis, cystitis). It's especially valuable for bladder infections, with antiseptic and antibacterial properties to fight E. coli, which clings to bladder walls. Chamomile also eases nausea and vomiting, and it relaxes muscle tension and digestive tract distress including pain, bloating, gas, constipation, and irritable bowel syndrome. It's a time-honored treatment for bronchial asthma, hay fever, and sinusitis.

CRANBERRY

Vaccinium macrocarpon, oxycoccos
PART USED: Berries

This red fruit is a remedy for urinary tract infections. Studies indicate that there are more than 50 million cases each year in the United States alone. Experts recommend cranberry juice and vitamin C to help urinary tract infections, but cranberry juice contains sugar, which supports bacteria, and it's only 10–30 percent cranberries. Cranberry tea is all cranberry, no sugar, and it comes with its own vitamin C. One of the ways that urinary tract infections are spread is from E. coli bacteria in the urethra moving up to the bladder, where it clings to the bladder lining. Women are more vulnerable, because their urethral canal is about seven inches shorter than a man's, and straighter. Cranberry comes to the rescue with two antioxidants, vitamins A and C. Studies show that cranberry prevents E. coli from clinging to bladder walls. Cranberry is also rich in calcium for strong bones and to prevent intestinal polyps, with iron for blood building, plus B-complex and essential minerals.

DONG QUAI

Angelica sinensis
PART USED: Root

This tea enhances your vital force, or chi. It's native to China, and a relative of *Angelica archangelica*, named for angels. Dong quai is known as *tang kuei* in China and has been a favored herb in Chinese medicinal blends for more than 2,000 years. It's known as a disbursing herb, one that can move stagnated body fluids to achieve more balance and harmony. It's also a disease fighter: antiviral, antifungal,

anti-inflammatory, antioxidant, and antirheumatic. It contains selenium—a natural barrier to disease—and it's rich in the antioxidant
vitamin E, with vitamin B_{12} for energy. It's a blood tonic with iron,
a vibrancy tea with silica, and a tea for tranquillity, with magnesium. It
helps to relieve constipation, it's a mild expectorant for chest congestion, and it's an excellent tea for menopausal women who don't want
estrogen risks, since dong quai has no estrogenic properties. It's also
a powerful source of nutrients to boost vitality; it helps to maintain
a healthy heart and build bone marrow to fight osteoporosis, which
are important concerns in menopause. It calms the nervous system
and eases stress. It stimulates circulation to enhance concentration
and memory, and it has antiaging virtues. It is also a good tea for
premenstrual tension, since it contains zinc and calcium, which are
often lacking in women who struggle with premenstrual syndrome.

Dong quai is exceptional for women, but herbalists recommended it as a tonic for both sexes to stabilize hormones and to increase energy and stamina. It also contains vitamins A, B_3, B-complex,
and C, sodium, phosphorus, potassium, silicon, coumarins, valeri-
anic acid (calming), and tannins.

ELDERBERRY

Sambucus nigra
PART USED: Berries

This berry tea is your first line of defense in flu season. It's a native
of Europe and Britain, with a long tradition as a remedy for colds,
coughs, the flu, and chest congestion. In Israel, elderberries are
combined with raspberries and citric acid for a flu remedy. It's for
respiratory conditions including hay fevers, allergies, colds, coughs,
tonsillitis, sore throats, and mouth infections. It removes mucus and
imbedded phlegm from the lungs to minimize allergic reactions that
cause hay fever, stuffiness, and tightness in the chest. Elder cleanses
the respiratory system and removes toxins from the body. It helps to

reduce fevers and inflammatory conditions. Historically, elder tea has been a cold remedy for children, and elderberry wine has been the adult cure in England. Among its vital properties are palmitic, linoleic, and linolenic acids, flavonoids (antioxidants), mucilage (for moistening), pectin, natural sugar, and a high content of vitamins A and C (strong antioxidants), which help to fight cancer.

FEVERFEW   *Chrysanthemum parthenium, Tanacetum parthenium*
PART USED: Leaves, Flowers, Stems

This member of the daisy family is a natural antihistamine that inhibits the release of histamines. High histamine levels in the blood have been linked to allergies, headaches, migraines, and depression. Studies show that feverfew works best to prevent recurring headaches and migraines when it is taken as a routine tea, instead of as a quick fix. Feverfew is also a decongestant to clear phlegm and relieve congestion in the chest and sinuses. It reduces tension to relieve bronchial spasms. It's also an anti-infammatory to fight all inflammatory conditions and diseases. In England, feverfew is used for arthritis and to ease the aches of sciatica and neuralgia. Feverfew also has bitters, which are healing to the digestive tract. It stimulates the production of digestive enzymes and strengthens the liver, which produces vital chemicals for digestion. Feverfew is soothing to the nerves and can be helpful for all nervous disorders and to ease tension. It's a soothing tea for premenstrual tension and irritability, and delayed periods.

GREEN TEA   *Camellia sinensis*
PART USED: Leaves

One of the earliest known medicinal herbs, *Camellia sinensis* was discovered in 2737 BC by the father of Chinese medicine, Emperor

Shen Nung. Legend says he was boiling water outdoors, a wind stirred, and green leaves fell into the water. He was enchanted by the fragrance and decided to taste the brew. From this discovery, the tea industry was born centuries later; green tea, jasmine, oolong, and black tea all originate from the same plant that Shen Nung discovered. Green tea is made from fresh-dried leaves of *Camellia sinensis*, jasmine is green tea with jasmine blossoms, oolong is made from mildly fermented dried leaves, and black, the most pungent, comes from fully fermented dried leaves of the same shrub.

The green tea seedlings were given as gifts from Chinese monks to Japanese monks. Today, green tea is known as the national beverage of Japan. It is generally agreed that fresh-dried leaves have more potent properties than do fermented leaves; therefore, green tea is the most medicinal, oolong is second, and black is third. However, all three have the same characteristics in different strengths.

Green tea contains polyphenols, which are powerful antioxidants that are 200 times stronger than vitamin E—equivalent to eating seven antioxidant vegetables. Anticancer catechins are also present in green tea, which protect the cells from carcinogens and toxins, fight free radical damage, and help to keep radioactive strontium 90 out of the bones. The catechins have shown the ability to inhibit or prevent the growth of cancer cells in in vitro studies. The catechins are also antibacterial and antiviral.

Green tea is a circulatory tonic, which helps to reduce cholesterol, lowers blood pressure, and prevents cardiovascular disease. It also helps to regulate blood sugar levels to fight diabetes. For respiratory problems, green tea is a bronchodilator, which opens the bronchial tubes for easier breathing. It is also a mild decongestant for bronchial congestion, vital for asthma and other respiratory weaknesses. Green tea contains fluoride for healthy teeth, and its polyphenols help to prevent gum disease and bacteria, which can lead to tooth decay and bad breath. A warm green tea bag on an inflamed or infected tooth can provide substantial relief from infection and pain while you call the dentist.

Green tea contains 40–50 milligrams of caffeine per cup, which is half the caffeine in a cup of coffee. It is available without caffeine, which makes it a less stimulating drink, more mellow in nature.

MILK THISTLE   *Silybum marianum*

PART USED: **Roots, Leaves, Seeds, Hulls**

This is an herb for renewal. It's a wholesome tea with a sweet nature, and it's a first-class remedy to fight toxins. Legend says that the white milky veins in milk thistle were created when Mary was nursing Jesus and some of her milk fell on the common thistle, giving the thistle white veins. Herbs that have sacred or spiritual associations often turn out to be herbs with special properties, and milk thistle is blessed with very special antioxidants for immune strength, liver renewal, and to bind toxins.

Milk thistle contains silymarin, a unique combination of flavonolignans (antioxidants) that protects liver cells from toxins and free radical damage. In German studies, liver poisons were tested against silymarin, and tests revealed that silymarin bound the toxins and fragmented others before they could damage the liver. Your liver plays a key role in immunity and health. It secretes bile, which stimulates digestive juices that break down nutrients from foods into absorbable forms that can be used by your cells for energy. It manufactures chemicals to detoxify the blood and remove pollutants and metabolic wastes. It helps to dissolve fat-soluble toxins, regulate proteins, and recycle hormones. When your liver is compromised, your whole system suffers. Silymarin is the only known natural compound that protects liver cells from damage and renews liver vitality, even in disease states. It's an excellent iced tea for recovery programs from alcohol or drugs and to protect the liver from harsh medications.

Common signs of liver weakness include recurring headaches, skin problems, depression, poor circulation, chronic fatigue, indigestion, irritability, mood swings, lack of concentration, diminished resistance to disease—which in turn, lead to premature aging. If you have one or more of these issues to resolve, add milk thistle tea to your daily routine. Milk thistle is also a natural antihistamine that represses the release of histamines in the body. High histamine levels in the blood are linked to allergies and headaches, and milk thistle combats both problems. Milk thistle is also an antidepressant. Studies show that milk thistle shows promise for treatment of prostate cancer, due to the toxin-fighting nature of silymarin.

Milk thistle can be a vital tea to use as a recovery treatment after chemotherapy and radiation. It is used in China as an adjunct to chemotherapy to insure minimal damage to the liver for cancer patients.

PEPPERMINT and SPEARMINT

Mentha piperita (Peppermint),
Mentha spicata (Spearmint)
PART USED: Whole Plant, Flowers

Peppermint is a tonic herb that is considered a cure-all. It's antiseptic, analgesic, and astringent, as well as a decongestant, pain reliever, and digestive aid with a calming nature; it strengthens the nervous system, eases stress and depression, and calms you all over. The menthol in oil of peppermint has an anesthetic effect on nerve endings in the stomach, which stops nausea and seasickness. One whiff of the fragrance is a pick-me-up. Taken as a tea, peppermint can ward off colds and infections, fight congestion in the chest, and clear nasal passages. It has been used for palpitations of the heart, colic, dyspepsia, and flatulence, and in baths to combat body odor. It has a healthy supply of nutrients that include the antioxidants vitamins A and C (flavonoids), B-complex, carotenoids, betaine, choline, minerals, tocopherols, phytol, azulene—and the vital oil of peppermint, which is the third most popular oil in the world after lemon and orange.

SPEARMINT: Most experts agree that spearmint is the mint that grew in the Holy Land and was mentioned in the Bible. The health virtues of spearmint are similar to peppermint, but milder.

ROSE HIPS

Rosa canina, rugosa, and centifolia
PART USED: Hips (dried fruit)

The rose's origins are believed to be thirty million years old. Legends say that all of the roses in the world bloomed when the Christ Child was born. The hips are the red coverings around the fruits, with a wealth of health benefits for young and old from skin to soul. The vital properties are so numerous, I have to list them: antibacterial, antidepressant, anti-inflammatory, antioxidant, antiseptic, antiviral, aphrodisiac, blood tonic, circulatory stimulant, cleanser, digestive aid, decongestant, free radical scavenger, infection fighter, hormone regulator, immunity booster, kidney tonic, phlegm remedy, recovery tonic, respiratory aid, skin hydration, support for adrenal glands, urinary tract cleanser.

See chapter 2, "Nature's Bouquet of Healing Herbs and Spices for Cooking" for the stories of saffron, fennel, and coriander, which are also used in the iced teas.

CHAPTER 23

Transforming Your Processed Foods

Don't Just Heat and Serve, Energize Them First!

You can transform processed foods into healthier fare with herbs and spices. It seems like a small step, but it can make a big difference in your health.

Pasta Sauce, Can or Jar

- Transform your processed sauce by heating it in a teaspoon of olive oil with fresh chopped garlic to burst the flavor. Add 1 teaspoon dried basil (or oregano) and 1 teaspoon of dried thyme to the sauce. Cover and let it simmer for a while, just like you'd do if you were making a fresh sauce. It will turn a processed sauce into something special.

- To enhance the nutritional value and add texture to your sauce, add fresh chopped mushrooms, onions, peppers, or your favorite vegetables.

- Turn your processed sauce into a thick and hearty meat sauce. Sauté ground beef in olive oil with fresh chopped garlic, thyme, basil, and/or oregano. Keep in mind that processed foods already contain lots of salt, so you don't need to add extra salt.

- Transform your processed sauce into a creamy cheese sauce by blending a cup of fat-free ricotta into the sauce, with ½ cup of fresh chopped parsley. You'll get a creamy cheese flavor that tastes like lasagna sauce, but it's lower in fat.

- To achieve a meat sauce flavor without adding meat, add 1–2 teaspoons of chile powder to a pasta sauce. Chile powder has a warming nature and lots of zest to give tomato sauce a real boost in flavor and energy.

Soups

Look at any can of soup as the base that you are going to transform into a rich, energizing soup. One can of your favorite soup can become the equivalent of two or three cans, with greater health benefits. To achieve this, you can:

1. Expand the liquid content with water or broth.

2. Add fresh or frozen vegetables that are similar to—or complementary to—the ones in the soup.

3. Add fresh or dried herbs and spices for flavor, energy, and healing power.

4. Add extra noodles or rice.

Other soup suggestions:

- Keep a selection of frozen mixed vegetables on hand to add to processed soups, to tide you over if you don't have fresh vegetables.

- Add ¼ cup chopped fresh celery, chives, or parsley to chicken-based soups for fresh green herbal energy with healing power.

- Add ¼ cup diced carrots for extra sweetness with antioxidant power.

- Add ¼ cup frozen turnips for a complementary vegetable for chicken-based soups. See chapter 12, "Veggie Versatility," to discover the health benefits of turnips.

- To cut the salt in chicken-based soups, expand the soup with water and make fresh egg noodles or rice to add to the soup.

- Transform your chicken soup into Chinese chicken soup by adding a teaspoon of fresh lemon juice and the white of one egg, whipped, just before serving.

- Hearty vegetables make vivid additions to beef-based soups. Add more water and shredded fresh carrots; chopped red, orange, or green peppers; ½ cup finely diced onions; fresh chopped garlic; cauliflower; leeks; or scallions. Keep a supply of frozen hearty vegetables on hand for beef-based soups.

- Beef-based soups can take on a deeper flavor with 1 teaspoon of allspice, chile powder, or coriander.

- To give beef-based soups a Middle Eastern flavor, try ½ teaspoon cumin or 1 teaspoon of turmeric, which helps to fight cancer and Alzheimer's.

- Add finely minced fresh parsley or chives to cream soups to wake up their flavor.

- Black bean soup can be enhanced with ½ cup diced plum tomatoes, fresh chopped garlic, cumin, and cinnamon.

Canned Beans

- Add 1 teaspoon dried coriander and ½ teaspoon cumin to create bean nectar.

- Expand the beans with chopped vegetables, or combine beans with ½ cup ground beef sautéed in olive oil and chopped garlic.

Frozen Dinners

- Remove frozen dinners from their cartons and cook them in glass oven bowls for better safety—since cartons can contain chemicals—and a better taste.

- Don't feel that frozen dinners are in an untouchable state. When heated, add fresh chopped parsley, minced garlic, chopped celery, or your choice of chopped vegetables to expand the dish with vital energy.

Frozen Fish

- Drizzle frozen fish with fresh lemon and your choice of an herb or spice before cooking. The green herbs are excellent on fish.

Top the fish with a fresh *Magic Teaspoon* topping, sauce, dip, or puree for fabulous energy.

Pouch Pastas

Turn any pouch pasta into a larger dish with more energy:

- Shells in creamy garlic sauce can become a healthier meal by adding a package of frozen spinach and a teaspoon of dill to the dish. What do you get? A creamy Florentine pasta with a pesto flavor. You also get a cost-effective dish that fits any budget. Pour it over sizzling steak tips, and you have a balanced meal in a flash.

- Pasta primavera: Add sliced red and yellow peppers, fresh chopped garlic, and chopped broccoli or peas to any creamy pasta in a pouch for a primavera.

- Other vegetables and herbs to add to pouch pastas: 1 cup shredded carrots, cooked in butter with a dash of allspice; 1 cup cauliflower (anticancer) steamed crisp.

- Revisit chapter 12, "Veggie Versatility," to find other vegetable recipes with herbs and spices to inspire you to expand your pouch pastas.

Boxed Macaroni and Cheese

- Expand the dish and energize it with vegetables, herbs, and spices. Macaroni and cheese can become a broccoli and cheddar dish with a garnish of parsley and a cup of broccoli. Simply expand the water you use, and cook the broccoli right in the mix.

- Macaroni and cheese can take on a different character every time you cook it, depending on the vegetables and herbs you use as enhancements.

Bottled Salad Dressings

- Freshen any processed salad dressing by adding a teaspoon of minced fresh parsley or chopped fresh garlic. It will wake up the flavor.

CHAPTER 24

Sugar Smarts

A New Outlook on Sugar Could Be Just What You Need

With herbs and spices as your allies, you can look at sugar from a whole new perspective—armed with support. Instead of focusing all of your energy on trying to cut sugar and feeling deprived, focus your attention on other important aspects of your menu that can give you pleasure without sugar surges. It's the winner's formula for living without routine glucose spikes that lift you up, only to let you down. It's based on getting steady, dependable energy.

Don't Eat Bland in Your Daily Menu

An important way to tame your urges for sweets is to add more herbs and spices to your daily menu. When your food has a rich, versatile flavor, and it provides vital nutrition for stable, long-term energy, you'll find more pleasure in your food, and you'll stay satisfied longer, which reduces your need to turn to sugary foods for satisfaction.

There are several herbs and spices that help to reduce your blood sugar level—like cayenne, celery seeds, cinnamon, coriander, dill, and garlic. There are many herbs and spices that are digestive aids to help you resolve common digestive disorders and stress—like anise, chives, fennel, ginger, horseradish, oregano, parsley, pepper, tarragon, and turmeric, and they have other fabulous health properties. All of the herbs and spices that improve your circulation also help to fight diabetes—including basil, mustard, rosemary, sage, and vanilla—and they also have other health properties to fight infections and diseases of aging. There are many herbs and spices that fight depression, which can lead you to sugar for a quick fix. Best of all, several herbs and spices are sweet—like cinnamon, anise, vanilla, and fresh basil. Put it all together in your menu with healthy food, and your everyday life is filled with pleasure and healing power. You get steady, dependable energy that won't let you down.

Don't Leave the House Hungry

Don't leave home in the morning with hunger on the rise. This is the best thing you can do to tame sugar urges throughout the day. Hunger is the body's call for nutrition; it's not a call for sweets. Many people respond to the hunger signal by turning to sugar-rich sweets for a quick lift and instant gratification, but the energy from sweets is short-lived. It's a quick surge in blood sugar, with empty calories that have no vitamins, minerals, or other nutrients to support your body's needs, and hunger surfaces again quickly, calling for nutrition.

What should you look for to satisfy your body's need for nutrition, and your need for pleasure when your hunger surfaces again? Look for something with fiber, enhanced with herbs and spices.

Fabulous Fiber: The Perfect Snack

Fiber helps to regulate your sugar absorption and stabilize sugar highs and lows. It also fills your stomach, which leads to a sense of satisfaction. The chew factor in fiber is also vital. It gets the process of digestion into full swing, which turns off your hunger signal in twenty minutes. Reach for a fiber snack with herbs and spices to wake up your senses, give you pleasure, and for immediate energy. A bland wheat cracker won't do the trick, but this recipe will invigorate you.

Tantalizing Trail Mix

When trail mixes first arrived in health stores, they were natural health blends of fiber and dried fruits, but look what's happened to them lately! Check the ingredients on the supermarket versions of packaged trail mixes. One of the first ingredients is sugar, corn syrup, or corn syrup solids. That means it's a maximized sugar mix, not a trail mix.

You need a trail mix that doesn't use sugar to get your attention. This trail mix will give you energy in an instant. Take a bag to work, leave one in your car, and keep a generous amount in a round, plastic, airtight container next to your computer to lift you out of slumps. It's a fabulous treat to meet hunger urges with lots of energy, nutrients, fiber, healing power, and satisfaction, instead of sugar surges.

This recipe makes 4 cups. Don't worry if you can't stop eating it, because fiber has a secondary benefit in addition to stabilizing your sugar absorption—it helps you store less fat. Fiber speeds up your food transit time—the time it takes for food to pass through your intestines. The longer food stays in your intestines, the more fat you can store as calories. The spicy blend of herbs and spices in this mix boosts your circulation and immunity and gives you a lift that will stay with you. I usually double this recipe, because it goes fast. It keeps you feeling young and vital.

>   3 cups wheat squares (unsugared)
>   1 cup Parmesan goldfish
>   ½ can smoked almonds
>   ⅛ cup butter
>
>   *Herb and Spice Mix*
>   ½ tablespoon Worcestershire sauce
>   ¼ teaspoon paprika
>   ¼ teaspoon dried thyme
>   ⅛ teaspoon black pepper (coarsely ground)
>   ⅛ teaspoon Tabasco sauce (or red hot cayenne pepper sauce)

Preparation. Preheat oven to 250 degrees. In large, shallow roasting pan, spread out wheat squares, goldfish, and almonds. In a separate pan, melt butter, add Herb and Spice Mix, and gently blend. Drizzle it over the cereal and stir to coat the cereal. Bake for 1 hour, gently stirring every 20 minutes. Cool the mix on a brown paper bag. Divide it into several sealed baggies. It's ready to go anywhere you go!

Rely on the Best Sweet Energy

Rely on natural fruits for your sweet treats, and you'll get sweetness in a health package. Sugar in fruit is naturally occurring sugar, the best kind of sugar, since it is an integral part of a food. In this form, sugar occurs naturally as part of a unit, which includes vitamins, minerals, enzymes, and fiber, and they all work together for your benefit. The fiber helps the sugar absorb with more blood glucose stability. The vitamins, minerals, and enzymes upgrade your health.

Frozen Blueberries and Grapes

Freeze blueberries and grapes in a plastic ziplock bag at home and at work. Feeling a slump coming on? Pop a frozen blueberry or grape in your mouth and let it defrost like an ice pop. They make energizing natural sugar snacks that wake you up in a flash.

Soft-Serve Sorbets

Freeze melon chunks and peach chunks in plastic ziplock bags. Toss them into a food processor or chopper, and blend. You get an instant soft-serve sorbet for a snack, with natural sugar and solid nutrition. You can add a dash of cinnamon or vanilla. That's healthy satisfaction.

Natural Applesauce

See the recipe for Natural Applesauce in chapter 7, "Breakfast Energy." It's a sweet treat you can turn to for steady, dependable energy, and apples are a wonder food.

Look for Sweet Treats with Herbs and Spices That Offset the Sugar That Is Used for Sweetness

Natural Licorice Bits

It's hard to believe that so much healing power could be in a sweet treat. Natural licorice bits contain two sweet herbs—extract of licorice and extract of anise—and natural molasses. Pop one in your mouth, and the sweetness lingers for hours. Licorice is a tonic for your adrenal glands, which helps you fight fatigue, depression, irritability, indigestion, poor nutrient assimilation, and lack of concentration. It's an ACE root herb that contains all three antioxidants—vitamins A, C, and E—with flavonoids that fight cancer and free radical damage. Licorice is also an excellent source of nutrients and an anti-inflammatory.

Anise is an aromatic herb that is also an anti-inflammatory, a pain reliever, and an antifungal. It's excellent for people with respiratory conditions, including asthma. Molasses is a cane concentrate that is only one-third sugar, with something sugar can't provide: vitamins and minerals, including calcium, iron, zinc, vitamin B-complex, magnesium, chromium, copper, and potassium. Natural licorice is available in health food stores.

Crystallized Ginger

Ginger is coated with crystallized sugar, but it's not a lot of sugar, and you get the powerful benefits of ginger in this sweet treat. Ginger has been a renowned root for more than 2,000 years. It's a heart herb with a warming nature that helps to lower your blood cholesterol, stabilize blood pressure, and reduce the risks of heart attacks and strokes. It's also an herb for weight control and digestion. It increases body heat, which helps to burn calories. It's cleansing and calming, and a circulatory stimulant.

This is an excellent treat to carry with you if you live in a cold climate and have to walk to the train or spend time outdoors. It warms you all over.

Crystallized ginger also comes chocolate-coated, and chocolate is a health food with antioxidant power to fight free radicals and degenerative diseases. It's an antiaging sweet treat. You can also make your own chocolate ginger. Buy the large, flat pieces of crystallized ginger, heat dark chocolate cooking bits in a saucepan, dip the crystallized ginger into the chocolate, and chill it for an hour to harden the chocolate.

Swedish Peppernut Cookies

See the recipe for Swedish Peppernuts in chapter 21, "Desserts from Cool to Sweet." Three great spices tame the sugar in these cookies—cardamom, cinnamon, and white pepper—and it's only a half cup of sugar for a recipe that makes fifty small cookies. Cardamom is pungent and warming, and it's a spirit lifter, a digestive aid, and calming for the central nervous system, which helps to reduce irritability, headaches, and nervous tension. Cinnamon is a sweet spice that fights bacteria, and viral and fungal infections, and it helps to reduce high blood pressure. Studies show it helps to reduce blood sugar levels to fight adult-onset diabetes. Pepper—the master spice—is hot, aromatic, and antibacterial to fight infections. It helps to burn fats, and it's a circulatory stimulant for energy.

Herbal Honey Spread on Crackers or Muffins

A half teaspoon of herb or spice honey on crackers or a muffin will satisfy your desire for sweetness with stable sugar absorption and fiber you need for dependable energy and fitness. Remember, honey is sweeter than sugar, so a little goes a long way.

FENNEL HONEY. Fennel has a soothing nature, and it's a marvelous herb for digestive strength.

CORIANDER SPICE HONEY is like a honey nectar. It's a spirit lifter and a real energizer.

ROSEMARY HONEY has a rich, piney taste. It stimulates circulation, enhances memory, and it's good for your heart.

SPEARMINT HONEY is a minty defense against colds, flu, and infections. It's a great honey snack for office environments that don't circulate fresh air.

ANISE HONEY is an extra-sweet honey; a natural anti-inflammatory and a time-honored honey for respiratory strength.

Rely on Fresh Iced Teas to Replace Colas, Sodas, and Fruit Drinks, the Ultra-Sugar Drinks

See chapter 22, "Magic Teaspoon Iced Teas," for recipes that rely on natural fruit sweetness and a taste of honey, which has antibacterial properties and many micronutrients, and absorbs with more stability than sugar.

Try This Sugar Experiment to Find Out How Much Sugar You Can Lose

If you drink two colas per day (or sodas, or sugared fruit drinks)—which have approximately 8 teaspoons of sugar in each soda (some have 10–12)—you are getting 16 teaspoons of extra sugar in one day, or 112 teaspoons of extra sugar in one week.

Take a bag of white sugar and put 112 teaspoons of white sugar in a jar. Look at it! That's a lot of extra sugar in your body in one week. Now, pour half of the sugar from your jar back into your sugar bag.

You can cut 56 teaspoons of sugar from your body in one week if you replace 1 cola, soda, or fruit drink with one *Magic Teaspoon* iced tea. That means that you will lose 224 teaspoons of sugar from your body in one month. Imagine putting 224 teaspoons of sugar in a jar—that's a lot of sugar you didn't eat! It's like money in the bank when it comes to your health, and your body will love you for it.

Check the ingredients label on your favorite cranberry juice. If the first ingredient isn't cranberry, but sugar, that means it's a sugar drink, not a fruit drink. *The Magic Teaspoon* tea Raz-a-ma-taz gives you pure, concentrated cranberry—which fights E. coli and infections. That's a cranberry drink you can count on for pure cranberry energy and stable sugar absorption.

Carry iced teas in a thermos to have them on hand when you're on the run and most susceptible to grabbing a quick cola, soda, or fruit drink. Take your Thermos to work, to the gym, or keep it in your car for long drives. Set your goal: Replace one cola, soda, or fruit drink with one iced tea to lose 224 teaspoons of sugar this month.

Get to Know the Big Sugar Boosters: Shake and Pour Sugars

We all use them—sauces, salad dressings, and prepared spreads that come in bottles or jars and are so easy to use—but some brands can be excessively high in sugar. You can make a stunning reduction in your weekly sugar intake if you substitute a few fresh versions for some of your shake and pour sugar sauces, dressings, and spreads. To make your label reading less troublesome, I did a little detective work for you:

Cocktail Sauces

Cocktail sauces can be sugar sauces! Here are the ingredients you might find on the labels of popular cocktail sauces, listed in order of appearance: tomato paste, corn syrups, vinegar, water, horseradish, salt, vegetable oil . . . two additional sugars might appear at the bottom after lemon juice, spices, additives, and preservatives. What can you do?

Use Roasted Red Pepper Puree (chapter 8) for your cocktail sauce—it's a burst of pleasure on shrimp or any white fish. The only sugar is the naturally occurring sugar that is present in red peppers, and the spices are deep and penetrating. You'll get a stunning reduction in sugar excess by replacing your cocktail sauce in a jar.

Salad Dressings

Salad Dressings can be sugar dressings! I found three different styles and brands of salad dressings that have the same essential ingredients on the label in different orders. Salad Dressing #1: Water, vegetable oil (soybean or canola), high fructose corn syrup, vinegar . . . Salad Dressing #2: Water, corn syrup, vinegar, whey . . . Salad Dressing # 3: Vinegar, water, high fructose corn syrup, vegetable oil . . . It's sugared water with oils and a few spices.

Look for salad dressings with sugar listed closer to the bottom of the list, or make Fresh Thousand Island Dressing, EZ Blue Cheese Dressing, or any fresh dressing like the ones in chapter 10. Keep them on hand for fresh salads, and you'll make another stunning cut in your sugar intake. Sugars and additives only blunt the flavor of herbs and spices in salad dressing blends, so you'll be getting a bonus of vivid flavors in fresh salad dressings—and that means pleasure.

Ketchup

Ketchup can be overwhelmed with sugar, and most people use it liberally. I found several brands that listed these ingredients: Tomato concentrate (water and tomato paste), high fructose corn syrup, corn syrup, vinegar, spices . . . The second ingredient can be high fructose corn syrup, followed by the third ingredient, corn syrup.

That's not ketchup, it's red high fructose corn syrup. I went to the kitchen, set out glass bowls with ketchup in one bowl and tomato paste in the other. This is the result:

✿ Fresh Ketchup

This recipe for ketchup is all energy, tomato flavor, and health power. Remember that tomatoes have lycopene, a cancer fighter, and a horseradish–mustard blend is a circulatory stimulant for tired blood, a digestive aid, and a cleanser for toxins in your body, and it strengthens blood vessels and helps to reduce high blood pressure. Tomatoes also contains vitamin C, an antioxidant that helps to fight infections, free radical damage, and diseases of aging. Isn't it a shame to smother all of that power with the empty calories of corn syrup sugars that have no nutrition, elevate your blood sugar, and make you less resistant to infections? The horseradish blend (without sugar) provides vinegar, some water, and spicy flavoring to this ketchup. To make a larger quantity of this recipe, adjust the blend upward. It retains its fresh taste for weeks in the refrigerator, and it's a health bonus from the outset. Jar it.

2 teaspoons tomato paste (without sugar)*	¼ teaspoon lemon pepper
1 teaspoon horseradish blend (without sugar)	Dash of paprika
	Dash of allspice
¼ teaspoon onion powder	¼–½ teaspoon honey (or honey spread) to taste
4–6 teaspoons of water to thin	

*Check the ingredients in tomato paste and mustard blends before you buy them. They can contain sugar or corn syrups as sweeteners as a surprise.

Preparation. Combine all ingredients and blend. Try it on a burger. You'll never miss the sugar, and your body will thank you for it.

Know Your Refined Sugars

Refined sugars are sugars that are removed from their source (the food) and increased in potency—often doubled. They're primarily used as sweeteners or ingredients in processing. Refined white sugar is the ingredient listed as sugar on food labels. It's high-potency sugar—half fructose and half dextrose—100 percent maximized. Corn syrups and high fructose corn syrups are maximized refined sugars with high-potency fructose and dextrose. Refined sugars can be the total content of the food, as is the case in cola, gummi bears, and jelly beans. Refined sugars are known as empty calories—all sugar calories, no nutrition. Stripped from its food source, refined sugar has no vitamins, minerals, nutrients, or fiber. Without fiber, refined sugars are absorbed quickly, and your blood glucose rises swiftly.

Limit the Use of Processed Foods for Main Meals

Processed foods have refined sugars added, and that spells *sugar excess* for the average consumer. Before we had processing—canning, drying, freezing, pickling, preserving, sweetening, coloring, and texturizing—sugar excess wasn't the problem it is today. Today, 70 percent of our foods are processed, and we have no control over the sugar content, since they are prepackaged and predetermined by standards we might not set for ourselves. Often, more than 400 calories per day can be eaten as empty calories from the sugar in processed foods. Those calories can be eaten in healthier ways—in fresh foods, to give you more pleasure and satisfaction, and more power for your calories.

Compare fresh pasta salad to a boxed pasta salad with a seasoning packet:

FRESH PASTA SALAD WITH VEGETABLES	BOXED PASTA SALAD WITH SEASONING PACKET
Fiber content is high	Fiber is stripped out
Fat content is low	Fat is added in
Simple sugars occur naturally	High-potency sugars are added
High vitamin and mineral content	Nutrition stripped out
Protein is intact	Protein is damaged in processing
Low calories overall	Empty calories (calories without nutrition)

Often processed foods will put some nutrition back in, but the amounts are negligible compared to fresh food, and they are not balanced the way real foods are balanced.

When your menu includes too many processed foods, you lose fiber for intestinal health, protein, vitamins, and minerals for strength, energy, and resistance to disease. Processed foods can be eaten in a flash, with no chewing and minimal salivation, and no time for hunger to abate naturally from chewing.

Focus Your Sugar Search to Seek Sugar on Labels

Instead of glancing at various labels on a random basis to check for sugar, identify the top five processed foods you use most frequently, such as spaghetti sauce. Compare the ingredients labels on different brands, and buy the brand that has the least amount of sugar—lowest on the list of ingredients. Don't be misled by marketing claims that distract you from the ingredients label.

The term "natural grain" on a cereal box might seem appealing, but the cereal can have six teaspoons of sugar in every cup. The grain is technically natural, but the volume of sugar used to sweeten the grain may be off the charts. The only way to know for sure is to check the ingredients label.

The term "lower in sugar" doesn't mean much, unless the product answers the question, lower than what? Lower than it was before? The sugar content can be lower than it was before in that particular food, but it can still appear first on the ingredients label, meaning that it's primarily a sugar food.

The terms "sugar-free" or "no sugar added" don't mean that there is no sugar in these foods. The sugar can come from artificial sweeteners known as sugar alcohols, which are often included in foods for "low-carb" diets. Sugar alcohols tend to have half the sweetness and half the calories of regular sugar, and tend to elevate blood sugar less dramatically than does regular sugar. The trouble is, people might think that "sugar-free" or "no sugar added" means there is no sugar in these foods, and they eat more of them, which can cause side effects, like stomach discomfort, bloating, and a laxative effect. If too many grams of sugar alcohols are consumed in one day, they can cause an elevation in blood sugar and diarrhea.

Rely on Ingredients Labels to Find the Sugar in Foods

Ingredients are listed by weight on food labels. The heaviest ingredient is listed at the top, and the lightest at the bottom.

NAMES OF SUGARS TO LOOK FOR ON THE LABEL: Sugar, corn syrup, corn syrup solids, caramel, dextrose, fructose, invert sugar, lactose, maltose, raw sugar, sucrose, turbinado.

NAMES OF SUGAR ALCOHOLS TO LOOK FOR ON THE LABEL: Glycerol, hydrogenated starch hydrolysates, inositol, isomalt, lactitol, mannitol, maltitol, maltitol syrup, sorbitol, starch hydrolysates, xylitol. More common in European foods: dithioerythritol, dulcitol, erythritol, galactitol, ribitol.

How Sweet Is It?

- If sugar is listed first on the ingredients label, the product is primarily sugar.

- If sugar is listed second or third, the product is still high in sugar.

- If two or three sugars are listed midway on the label, the product is still high in sugar.

- If sugar is listed near the bottom, it's the best version.

The search for the perfect sugar in the modern world is never-ending. New artificial sweeteners arrive every day. Artificial sweeteners will be listed by name somewhere on the food, but not necessarily on the ingredients label. Some work well, and others don't. Do a Web search on your favorite artificial sweetener by name. It will exercise your sugar smarts.

In the world of artificial sweeteners, the quest for a perfect sugar is defined this way: a sweet taste and absorbable sugar that doesn't raise blood glucose levels unnaturally high, with less calories than refined or processed sugar.

What might that perfect sugar be?

We already have one. It's a fruit.

Strictly speaking, an orange is perfect sugar. It has a sweet taste and absorbable sugar that doesn't raise blood glucose levels unnaturally high—with less calories than refined white or processed sugar. It also comes in a health package that includes vitamins, minerals, antioxidants, and lots of energy. Enjoy an orange to get the taste of a perfect sugar. Combine it with a spice that helps to lower your blood sugar and fights infections, and you've got everything you need in a sweet dessert.

🌿 Orange Segments Dipped in Creamy Orange Nectar Dressing

See the recipe for Creamy Orange Nectar Dressing in chapter 10, "Sumptuous Green Salads and Fresh Dressings."

When you use herbs and spices freely in your recipes, like the *Magic Teaspoon* recipes do, the flavor of the herbs and spices will work their own magic, gradually retraining your palate to enjoy rich tastes that don't need excess sugar to get your attention.

Then one day, you'll notice that you crave drinks that aren't excessively sweet; you crave fresh foods because they make you feel more energized. You'll start to notice how much sugar there is in most processed foods and drinks, and you won't even think of them as conveniences anymore. That day, you'll realize that your palate has been retrained to enjoy subtle tastes and crave less sugar.

That's when you have it beat.

Bon Appetit!

BIBLIOGRAPHY

Ahmad N., D. K. Feyes, A. L. R. Nieminen, Mukhtar H. Agarwal. "Green Tea Constiutent Epigallocatechin-3 gallate and Induction of Apoptosis and Cell Cycle Arrest in Human Carcinoma Cells." *Journal of the National Cancer Institute* 89 (1997):1881–1886.

Barney, Paul D. "The Cranberry Cure." *Herbs for Health* November/December 1996.

Bentley, Virginia Williams. *Let Herbs Do It.* Boston, MA: Houghton Mifflin, 1973.

Brooks, Svevo, ed. *The Protocol Journal of Botanical Medicine.* Ayer, MA: Herbal Research Publications.

Burton Goldberg Group. *Alternative Medicine: The Definitive Guide.* Fife, WA: Future Medicine Publishing, Inc.

Chevallier, Andrew. *The Encyclopedia of Medicinal Plants.* New York: DK Publishing.

Chew, Robin. "Charlemagne King of the Franks and Emperor of the Holy Roman Empire 742–814." Lucid Interactive. http://www.lucidcafe.com/library/96apr/Charlemagne.html.

Child, Julia. *Mastering the Art of French Cooking,* vol. 2. New York: Alfred A. Knopf, 1970.

Clendinnen, Inga. "Imperial City of the Aztecs: Mexico-Tenochtitlan." Common-place. *The Interactive Journal of Early American Life.* http://www.common-place.org/vol-03/no-04/mexico-city.

Dunne, Lavon J. *Nutrition Almanac,* 3rd ed. New York: McGraw-Hill.

Farrell, Nicholas. "Tradition—Zest for Life." Waitrose Food Illustrated. http://www.waitrose.com/food_drink/wfi/foodissues/foodsafety scienceandhealth/

Farwell, Edith Foster. *A Book of Herbs.* Piermont, NY: The White Pine Press.

Foley, Daniel J. *Herbs for Use and Delight: An Anthology from the Herbarist.* New York: The Herb Society of America, Dover Publications, 1971.

Foster, Steven. "Fighting Depression the Herbal Way." *Herbs for Health* November/December 1996.

German Federal Institute for Drugs and Medical Devices Commission E, et al. *The Complete German Commission E Monographs: Therapeutic Guide to Herbal Medicines.* Austin, TX: American Botanical Council, 1998.

Greenwald, John. "Herbal Healing." *Time* November 23, 1998.

Grieve, M. *A Modern Herbal,* edited by C. F. Leyel. New York: Hufner Press, Div. of Macmillan Publishing.

Herb Research Foundation: "Extra-Virgin Is the Oil of Choice to Protect Against LDL Oxidation: Olive Oil (*Olea europea*)." Herb World News Online. http://www.herbs.org/current/olivechoice.htm.

Hobbs, Christopher. *Handbook for Herbal Healing.* Santa Cruz, CA: Botanica Press.

Hudson, J. L. *The Ethnobotanical Catalog of Seeds.* La Honda, CA: J. L. Hudson, Seedsman. http://www.jlhudsonseeds.net/Catalog.htm.

Jarvis, D. C. *Folk Medicine.* New York: Ballantine Books, Div. of Random House.

Jellicoe, Geoffrey, Susan Jellicoe, Patrick Goode, and Michael Lancaster. *The Oxford Companion to Gardens.* New York: Oxford University Press, 1986.

Khafif, A., S. P. Schants, T. C. Chou, et al. "Quantitation of chemopreventive synergism between (-)-epigallocatechin- 3-gallate and curcumin in normal, premalignant and malignant human oral epithelial cells." *Carcinogenesis* 19 (1998): 419–424.

King, Ronald. *The Quest for Paradise.* New York: Mayflower Books, 1979.

Knighthood, Chivalry, and Tournaments Resource Library. "Charlemagne the King: An Biography from Will Durant's *Story of Civilization* 1950." http://www.chronique.com/Library/MedHistory/charlemagne .htm.eborder.

Kumar, P. Vinoid, and Shyama Rajagopal. "Researchers Find Tea a Healthy Drink." http://www.indianexpress.com/fe/daily.

Kuts-Cheraux, A. W. *Naturae Medicina and Naturopathic Dispensatory.* Yellow Springs, OH: American Naturopathic Physicians and Surgeons Association, Antioch Press.

Lowe, Carl. "Natural Mood Boosters." *Energy Times* November/December 1997.

Marion, Joseph B. *Anti-Aging Manual: The Encyclopedia of Natural*

Health. Woodstock, CT: Information Pioneers.

McIntyre, Anne. *The Complete Woman's Herbal.* New York: Henry Holt.

Medicinal Spices Exhibit, UCLA Biomedical Library, History & Special Collections. http://unitproj.library.ucla.edu/biomed/spice/index.cfm?displayID=21

OMindell, Earl. *Herb Bible.* New York: Simon and Schuster.

Morton, M. S., et. al., "Lignans and Isoflavonoids in Plasma and Prostatic Fluid in Men: Samples From Portugal, Hong Kong, and the United Kingdom." *Prostate* (1997).

Mowrey, D. B., and D. E. Clayson. "Motion Sickness, Ginger and Psychophysics." *Lancet,* March 1982.

Mowrey, Daniel. *Herbal Tonics and Therapies.* Avenel, NJ: Wings Books, Div. of Random House.

Ody, Penelope. *The Complete Medicinal Herbal.* New York: Dorling Kindersley.

Oldenburger-Ebbers, Carla S. "Introduction to Dutch Gardens and Garden Architecture." Wageningen UR. http://library.wur.nl/speccol/intro.html.

Rago, Linda Ours. *Dooryard Herbs.* Shepherdstown, WV: Carabelle Books, 1984.

Ramirez-Tortosa, M. G. Urbano, M. Lopez-Jurado, et al. "Extra-Virgin Olive Oil Increases the Resistance of LDL to Oxidation More Than Refined Olive Oil in Free-Living Men with Peripheral Vascular Disease." *The Journal of Nutrition* 129 (1999):2177–2183.

Rector-Page, Linda G. *Healthy Healing.* Sonora, CA: Healthy Healing Publications.

Reid, Daniel. *The Tao of Health, Sex and Longevity.* New York: Simon & Schuster.

Rose, Jeanne. *Modern Herbal.* New York: Perigee Books.

Schardt, David. "Herbs for the Nerves." *Nutrition Action Health Letter* 25, no. 8, October 1998.

Strawberry Banke. "A Collection of Plants Grown in New England Before 1800: The Herb Garden at Strawberry Banke Museum." http://www.strawberrybanke.org/museum/herb/herb.html.

The Epicentre. "Encyclopedia of Spices." http://www.theepicentre.com/Spices/vanilla.html.

Tillery, Carolyn Quick. *The African-American Heritage Cookbook.* NJ: Carol Publishing Group, 1991.

Tyler, V. E. *Herbs of Choice: The Therapeutic Use of Phytomedicinals.* New York: Hayworth Press.

Wallace, Edward C. "Arthritis Pain Relief." *Energy Times* February 1998.

Weil, Andrew. *Spontaneous Healing.* New York: Alfred A. Knopf, Inc.

Weinberger, Stanley. *Candida Albicans: The Quiet Epidemic.* Larkspur, CA: Healing Within Products.

Welker, Glenn. "The Aztecs/Mexicas." Indians.org. http://www.indians.org/welker/aztec.htm.

Wren, R. C. *Potter's New Cyclopaedia of Botanical Drugs and Preparations.* New York: Pitman Publishing Corporation.

Z. Reina, Elisa L., Andrea G. "The Hanging Gardens of Babylon." http://www.angelfire.com/ny/anghockey/hanginggardens.html.

Zajaczkowa, Jadwiga (Jennifer Heise). "Medieval and Renaissance Gardens." Jadwiga's Herbs Homepage. http://www.gallowglass.org/jadwiga/herbs/medievalgardens.htm.